ESSENTIALS OF
PREVENTIVE MEDICINE

ESSENTIALS OF PREVENTIVE MEDICINE

J. A. MUIR GRAY
MD, MRCGP, MRCP (Glas)
Community Physician
Oxfordshire Health Authority

GODFREY FOWLER
BM, FRCGP, DCH, DRCOG
General Practitioner, Oxford
Clinical Reader in General Practice
University of Oxford

BLACKWELL SCIENTIFIC PUBLICATIONS

OXFORD LONDON EDINBURGH

BOSTON PALO ALTO MELBOURNE

© 1984 by
Blackwell Scientific Publications
Editorial offices:
Osney Mead, Oxford, OX2 0EL
8 John Street, London, WC1N 2ES
9 Forrest Road, Edinburgh, EH1 2QH
52 Beacon Street, Boston
Massachusetts 02108, USA
706 Cowper Street, Palo Alto
California 94301, USA
99 Barry Street, Carlton
Victoria 3053, Australia

First published 1984

Set by Oxprint Ltd, Oxford
and printed and bound
in Great Britain by
William Clowes Limited,
Beccles and London

DISTRIBUTORS

USA
Blackwell Mosby Book Distributors
11830 Westline Industrial Drive
St Louis, Missouri 63141

Canada
Blackwell Mosby Book Distributors
120 Melford Drive, Scarborough
Ontario, M1B 2X4

Australia
Blackwell Scientific Book
Distributors
31 Advantage Road, Highett
Victoria 3190

British Library
Cataloguing in Publication Data

Gray, Muir
Essentials of preventive medicine.
1. Medicine, Preventive
I. Title II. Fowler, Godfrey
614.4'4   RA425

ISBN 0-632-01044-4

CONTENTS

Common Health Problems

PREVENTING DISEASE

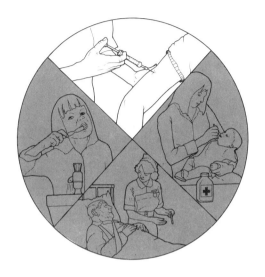

CHAPTER 1
THE SCOPE FOR PREVENTION

Unless every birth and every death is sedulously recorded it is impossible to calculate changes in the birth rate, the death rate, the expectation of life, or any other demographic trend. It is therefore impossible to know about changes in mortality rates which might have taken place before the notification of all births and deaths was required by law. However, medical and economic historians have adopted ingenious means of assessing population changes and, using sources such as registers compiled for the purposes of taxation, it is possible to calculate changes in the size of the population in times past. The increase in the population that has occurred owes more to the cumulative effect of human fertility than to a decline in mortality, but there is evidence that the mortality from certain diseases declined long before any effective preventive measures were introduced: for example, there were epidemics of typhus in Britain in 1718, 1728 and 1951, each following a bad harvest, and the disease then waned as the food supply improved; leprosy was once common in Europe but vanished before any effective preventive or curative measures were available; and plague vanished from Europe for no known reason.

Some diseases were therefore prevented but it seems that the only preventive measure that had any effect before the nineteenth century was an increase in food supply, and this can scarcely be called preventive medicine for the principal objectives of those who were improving food supply were not medical objectives but those two enduring motives—greed and fear of starvation.

Nineteenth century

Mortality in Britain began to fall in about 1870 (Fig. 1.1). Although death certificates of the time were often inaccurate because of mistaken diagnosis and carelessness in their completion, it is

3

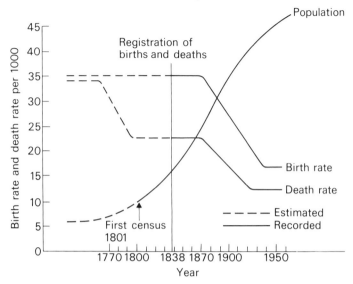

Fig. 1.1. Birth and death rates in the population of England and Wales from 1700 to 1900. (After McKeown, T. & Lowe, C. R. (1974) *An Introduction to Social Medicine*. Basil Blackwell, Oxford.)

possible to identify the diseases which declined during this period. There is no doubt that the predominant reason for this reduction was a decline in infectious diseases, but there is less certainty about the factors responsible. Professor Thomas McKeown has suggested that the decline in tuberculosis mortality was the most important single cause but that a number of other diseases also became less widespread (Fig. 1.2).

Means of prevention

Any decline in mortality such as that shown in Fig. 1.2 or the fall in coronary mortality which has recently occurred in the U.S.A. can be analysed by asking four questions.

1 Is this a real decline or just a change in the way people recorded or collected statistics?

2 Has there been a natural biological change in either the factor causing the disease or in the people who are at risk?

3 Have any effective treatments been introduced?

4 Have any effective preventive measures been introduced?

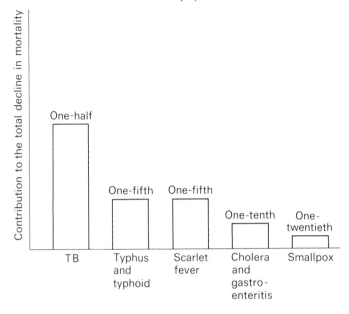

Fig. 1.2. Relative importance of different diseases to the total decline in mortality.

Having accepted that there was a real decline in mortality from infectious diseases it is appropriate to ask the other three questions to try to determine its causes (Table 1.1).

The decline in mortality from infections which has occurred in all developed countries can therefore be explained, but there is another important question which has to be asked: Why were these measures introduced in Britain in the middle of the nineteenth century; why not in the middle of the eighteenth or, for that matter, in the middle of the twentieth century? The answer to this question, the real historian's question, takes us from the practicalities of civil engineering into the realms of politics.

Politics of prevention

The preventive measures described in the previous section were introduced by law, but why did the legislators decide to act when they did? A number of social and political changes can be identified in countries which have introduced these public health services. These are the political prerequisites for preventive medicine, and can be summarized under the following points.

Table 1.1. Possible causes for a decline in mortality and their application to the nineteenth century.

Reason for decline in mortality	Relevance to nineteenth century decline in mortality
Was there a change in the natural history of these diseases, either a change in the susceptibility of the host or the virulence of the infecting micro-organism?	Man could not evolve quickly enough for genetic changes to reduce his susceptibility. Bacteria and virus can mutate much more quickly but it is thought that this is only relevant to the decline in the mortality from scarlet fever
Were any effective treatments introduced?	Not relevant. Most of the decline in mortality was due to the prevention of disease
Were any effective preventive measures introduced?	
Provision of pure water and official disposal of sewage	Decrease in number of people infected by bacteria causing typhoid, cholera, dysentery and diarrhoea
Better nutrition	Increased resistance to infection with tuberculosis and typhus, increased ability to recover from all types of infections
Better housing	Reduced spread of typhus and tuberculosis
Vaccination	Effective only for smallpox prevention

1 Scientific knowledge was influential. Legislation on water and sewage was introduced in Britain before the bacteria causing typhoid and cholera were discovered. Nevertheless, the knowledge that such diseases spread in water and not in the air was an important nineteenth century breakthrough.

2 Increasing wealth due to industrialization and trade allowed the public works to be done.

3 Fear was important. Consider the impact that 30 000 cases of rabies would have in Britain or Australia today and try to imagine the impact of cholera in Europe in 1831, the year of the first great epidemic. Furthermore, cholera and typhoid affected rich and poor so the legislators were afraid.

4 Poor people became better organized and educated, and were able to argue for improved working and living conditions.

5 Philanthropic attitudes became more widespread and the numbers of rich people who were sympathetic towards, or actually campaigned for, social reforms increased.

6 The establishment of a competent bureaucracy and efficient systems of communication and control allowed laws to be implemented.

The relative importance of these trends is a matter for debate but all appear to have been important and the same changes are needed in many developing countries before their governments will introduce the necessary public health measures to prevent disease (see p. 206).

Politics of child health

Infant and child mortality rates did not begin to fall until about 1900, 30 years after the decline in adult mortality rates, and the reason why the necessary changes were not introduced until the turn of the century were primarily political. Indeed it could be argued that the principal motive for improving child health in Britain was fear of Germany, best demonstrated by a comparison of the political situation at the time with the health services subsequently introduced.

Political reasons for increased interest in child health

1892 Tirpitz appointed Secretary of State for the German Navy.

1899 Tirpitz introduced Naval Bill asking for money to build battleships. Fear of Germany grows.

1899 War Office in Britain becomes alarmed because many young men are medically unfit when examined at Boer War recruiting offices.

1900 Germany passes Supplementary Naval Act, with Reichstag support for Tirpitz. Fear in Britain increased by German support of Boers.

1902 Invasion fever in Britain; publication of *The Riddle of the Sands* causes widespread alarm.

1904 Inter-Departmental Committee on Physical Deterioration reports on reasons for 'the large percentage of rejections for physical causes of recruits for the Army'.

Services introduced
1902 Midwives Act—improvements in care for pregnant women.
1906 Education (Provision of Meals) Act—school meals provided.
1907 Education Act—school health service launched.
Development of health visiting service.

Epidemiological reasons for resultant decrease in deaths
Prevention of malnutrition halted the cumulative effects of malnutrition and infections such as measles.
Decline in gastroenteritis due to the prevention of gastrointestinal infections, better hygiene and safer care of affected children.

Twentieth and twenty-first centuries

The first half of the twentieth century saw the consolidation of these measures and the introduction of immunization, which has accelerated the decline in importance of infectious diseases and a change in the pattern of disease (Fig. 1.3).

New patterns of disease
The major challenge in the developed countries is now prevention of non-communicable diseases, e.g. in Britain, only three types of non-communicable disease were responsible for 50% of the life expectancy years lost in the 1970 s (Table 1.2).

Prevention of morbidity
Avoiding premature death is only one objective of prevention: it is equally important to identify and try to prevent diseases which cause suffering and disability. The use of hospital beds is one measure of morbidity and if studied it is found that the non-communicable diseases which cause suffering differ from those which cause loss of life. Three types of disorder again account for more than half the problem, but this time mental illness and mental handicap are in the top three and cancer and ischaemic heart disease are lower in the league table (Table 1.3).

   Other measurements of non-fatal diseases are (i) the reasons for general practitioner consultations, (ii) sickness absence from

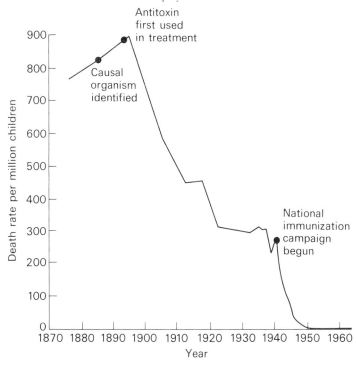

Fig. 1.3. Mean annual death rate from diphtheria of children under 15 years in England and Wales from 1870 to 1965. (After McKeown, T. & Lowe, C. R. (1974) *An Introduction to Social Medicine*. Basil Blackwell, Oxford.)

work and (iii) the use of out-patient services (Table 1.4). If these are added to the measures of the loss of life and use of hospital beds the total burden created by different types of disease can be calculated (Table 1.4). This pattern of disease presents a new challenge for prevention.

Scope for prevention
One method of estimating the scope for preventing premature deaths is to compare the mortality rates of one country with those of another, e.g. comparing the U.K. with Sweden and calculating the number of deaths which would have occurred in the U.K. if its mortality rates had been as low as the mortality rates in Sweden (Fig. 1.4).

Chapter 1

Table 1.2. Percentage of lost years of life expectancy due to different types of disease. (After Black,D. A. K. & Pole, J. D. (1975) *Brit. J. Soc. Prev. Med.* **29**, 222–7.)

Disease category	Percentage
Ischaemic heart disease	21.51
Neoplasms	20.63
Cerebrovascular disease	10.68
Other cardiovascular disease	8.74
Respiratory infections	7.11
Accidents and suicide	6.51
Bronchitis and asthma	4.10
Peripheral vascular disease	3.39
Congenital anomalies	3.17
Digestive disorders	2.48
Other respiratory diseases	1.54
Neurological disorders	1.41
Hypertension	1.30
Rheumatic heart disease	1.27
Cumulative burden of ranked categories	93.84
Unaccounted burden	5.54

Table 1.3. Percentage of total number of hospital beds used in England and Wales due to different types of disease. (After Black, D. A. K. & Pole, J. D. (1975) *Brit. J. Soc. Prev. Med.* **29**, 222–7.)

Disease category	Percentage
Mental illness	31.31
Mental handicap	15.19
Cerebrovascular disease	4.86
Malignant neoplasms	4.18
Digestive disorders	3.80
Childbirth	3.69
Accidents and suicide	3.44
Peripheral vascular disease	2.43
Neurological disorders	2.14
Ischaemic heart disease	2.11
Other cardiac diseases	2.06
Cumulative burden of ranked categories	75.21
Unaccounted burden	6.31

Table 1.4. Percentage contribution of different types of disease to the total burden of disease in England and Wales. (After Black, D. A. K. & Pole, J. D. (1975) *Brit. J. Soc. Prev. Med.* **29**, 222–7.)

Disease category	Indices mainly affected*	Percentage
Mental illness and handicap	1 2 3 4	13.60
Respiratory disease	3 4	13.47
Ischaemic heart disease	4 5	6.59
Bone and joint disease	2 3 4	6.38
Accidents and suicide	2 3 4	6.25
Neoplasms	5	6.08
Digestive disorders	2 3 4	4.56
Neurological disorders	2	4.11
Cerebrovascular disease	1 5	3.74
Skin diseases	2 3	2.55
Urogenital disease	2	2.31
		69.64

*1. in-patient days; 2. out-patient referrals; 3. GP consultations; 4. days of sickness benefit; 5. mortality as loss of life expectancy.

More than two countries can be compared in this way by identifying the lowest mortality rate for each age group from among all the countries and then calculating the number of deaths that would occur in each country if mortality rates in all its age groups were equal to the lowest mortality rate for each group. In Fig. 1.5 Sweden, the U.S.A., the U.K. and Canada are compared in this way so that the opportunities for health improvement can be estimated. Even in Sweden there is scope for prevention.

Effects of prevention—survival of the unfittest?
There has not been a significant increase in life *span* although there has been a significant increase in life *expectancy*. The curve of deaths shown in Fig. 1.6 is composed of two separate curves (broken lines)—the curve for premature deaths and the curve for senescent deaths. The effect of modern medicine, both preventive and curative, has been to make the curve of deaths taller, narrower and more symmetrical but not to shift it to the right.

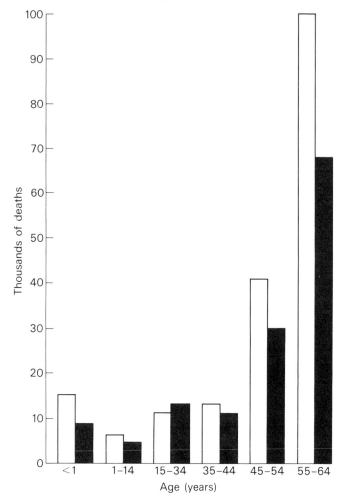

Fig. 1.4. Actual deaths (□) at ages 0–64 years in the U.K. (1972) and the number expected (■) if the corresponding Swedish death rates had applied to the U.K.

The increase in life expectancy may merely postpone the period of terminal disability and dependency on other people; it may even increase it. There is, however, another possibility— that the period of terminal disability and dependency is actually being reduced (Fig. 1.7). There are undoubtedly more disabled people in society because there are more old people, but there is

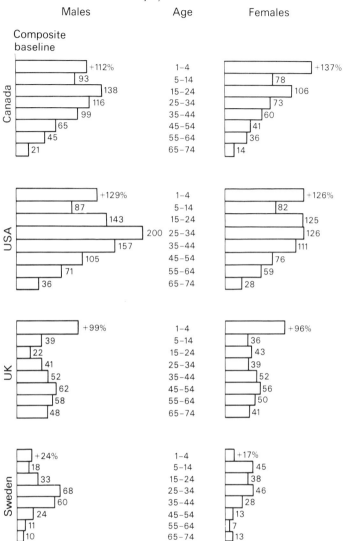

Fig. 1.5. Age/sex mortality rates in Canada, U.S.A., U.K. and Sweden, compared with composites of the lowest mortality rates found among the same four countries.

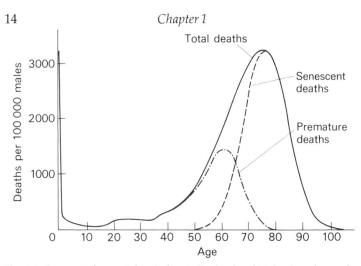

Fig. 1.6. Prospects for mortality decline in England and Wales, based on male deaths during 1950–52. (After Benjamin, B. & Overton, E. (1981) *Population Trends*, Spring 1981, 21–28.)

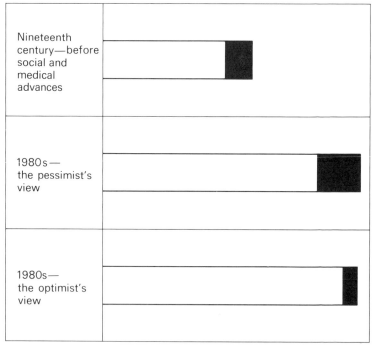

Fig. 1.7. Effects of social and medical advances on the number of active years (□) and the number of years of terminal dependency (■).

some evidence to suggest that the proportion of old people who are disabled is lower now than it was 40 years ago.

The data that are available are scanty and difficult to interpret but an increasing number of people are taking the optimistic view of the effects of medical and social advances. For this development is not, of course, solely due to the effects of modern medicine; it is the end result of a number of different trends. For example, the improvement in child health which took place in the early years of the century means that older people today are fitter than older people were 20 or 30 years ago.

Sir Richard Doll has said that his objective is 'to die young as late as possible' and it now appears that preventive medicine does not facilitate the survival of the unfittest. Its effects are to prevent disability as well as preventing premature death.

CHAPTER 2
THE PRACTICE OF PREVENTIVE MEDICINE

Clinical medicine is practised in hospitals, clinics, surgeries and in the patient's own home by nurses, doctors, occupational and physiotherapists and a host of other professionals. The practice of preventive medicine is even more difficult to describe briefly but the range of activities that contribute to the prevention of disease may be grouped under two rubrics—environmental and personal.

Environmental measures modify the environment in which an individual lives to reduce his risk of injury and disease. They may be divided into two types depending on whether they are designed to:
1 change the physical environment;
2 modify the social environment.
Personal preventive measures may also be subdivided into two types.
1 Those which are designed to change the individual's actions by health education.
2 Those services which have been developed specifically to reduce the risk of particular diseases. These are the personal preventive services, e.g. immunization, cervical cytology, the examination of all pregnant women to detect those whose fetus may be impaired, and family planning services.

It is, however, misleading to represent these four types of preventive measure on a family tree as shown in Fig. 2.1 for they are closely interwoven; e.g. the prevention of diseases caused by cigarette smoking requires, *inter alia*, education of individuals about the dangers of smoking and about the means the tobacco industry uses to influence the choices of young people. This makes it easier to introduce political measures to control cigarette advertising and to increase the price of cigarettes. Education of non-smokers about passive smoking facilitates changes in the physical environment, such as an increase in the provision of areas in which smoking is not allowed. This trend follows a

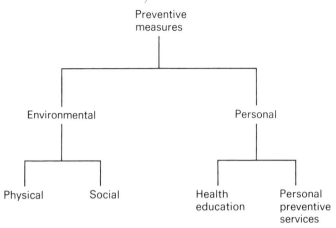

Fig. 2.1. Family tree of preventive medicine.

change in social attitudes, but it also helps to change social attitudes and this, in turn, makes it easier for the person who wishes to stop smoking to succeed. Therefore, the relationship between these four measures is more accurately represented by a Venn diagram than by a family tree (Fig. 2.2).

In the remainder of this chapter we will concentrate on those measures which are intended to change the physical and social environment in which the individual lives. Health education and personal preventive services will be covered in Chapters 3 and 7.

Physical environment

To reduce the risks to health in the physical environment requires a continuous process of control and surveillance (Fig. 2.3), as demonstrated by the following example. In the 1970s it was recognized that a number of children were being scalded by electric kettles. An analysis of these accidents revealed that some accidents were caused by the kettle being carried by the child but a number of design faults were also identified. Prototypes were tested in a laboratory and the resulting information was given to the industry and the Government.

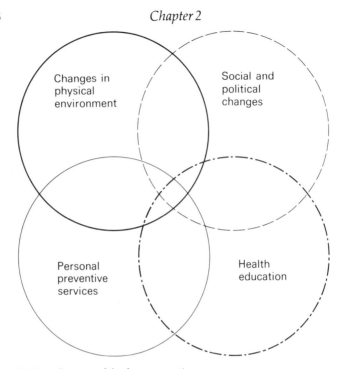

Fig. 2.2. Venn diagram of the four preventive measures.

Personal environment

Each individual has his own environment which consists of:
1 the water he drinks;
2 the air he breathes;
3 the food he eats;
4 the house he lives in;
5 the machines he uses;
6 the car he drives;
7 the place he works in;
8 the places where he plays and enjoys himself.
We can now consider the first five points in greater detail.

Water

Main health hazards
In developed countries, spread of infection by drinking water is very rare. New problems are:

(i) high concentrations of nitrates can cause difficulties in infants;

(ii) soft water may be a contributory cause of heart disease.

Typical protective measures
Control of industrial and agricultural effluent.
Maintenance of effective systems of sewage disposal.
Regular servicing of mains and sewers.

Typical monitoring programme
Regular chemical and bacteriological analysis of water samples.

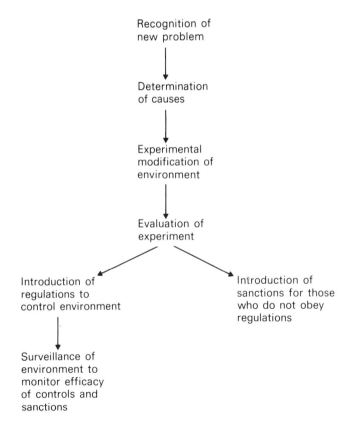

Fig. 2.3. Continuous process of control and surveillance of the physical environment.

Principal responsible authorities
Water authorities.
Department of the Environment.

Examples of legislative control
Control of Pollution Act (1974). Part III deals with 'control of entry of polluting matter and effluents into . . . rivers and coastal waters'.
Schedule 2 of the Act specifies the penalties, which include imprisonment.

Air

Main health hazards
Particulate pollution no longer a major problem except in certain areas. New problems are:
   (i) lead;
  (ii) sulphur dioxide;
 (iii) large numbers of new chemicals produced by industry.

Typical protective measures
Control of industrial and domestic emissions.
Modification of composition of petrol and design of engines.
Construction of high chimneys.

Typical monitoring programme
Regular sampling of air with analysis of particulate matter and chemicals.

Principal responsible authorities
Environmental Health Department of District Council.
Department of the Environment.

Examples of legislative control
Control of Pollution Act (1974) reinforces the Clean Air Act (1956) which allows the introduction of 'smoke control areas'.
Part IV of the Control of Pollution Act regulates the composition of motor fuels and the sulphur content of engine fuel.

Food

Main health hazards
Chemical contamination during growth, production or packaging.
Bacterial contamination during production, packaging or cooking.
Attention now being given to links between salt concentration and high blood pressure (see. p. 110).

Typical protective measures
Regulations on use of sprays and chemicals in plant and animal growth.
Pre-employment screening of food handlers to detect carriers of salmonella with surveillance of staff once in post.
Regulations on maximum concentrations of artificial chemicals, e.g. flavours, in food.
Investigation of reported cases and outbreaks of food poisoning.

Typical monitoring programme
Quality control by food industry—this is a good example of enlightened self-interest.

Principal responsible authorities
Environmental Health Departments of District Councils.
Public analysts.
Community physicians.
Ministry of Agriculture, Fisheries and Food.
European Parliament.

Examples of legislative control
Food and Drugs Act (1955) is the main Act covering the production, distribution and sale of food. Details of the controls are contained in Government papers called 'Statutory Instruments', e.g. the Milk and Dairies (General) Regulations (1959) or the Public Health (Shellfish) Regulations (1934).

Housing

Main health hazards
Very difficult to establish direct causal links between bad housing
and specific diseases because other factors, e.g. unemployment
and poverty, often affect people who are poorly housed. However, housing problems are associated with:
   (i) depression;
  (ii) anxiety;
 (iii) respiratory infections;
  (iv) difficulties in bringing up children;
   (v) home accidents;
  (vi) gastroenteritis, if water or sewage defective;
 (vii) handicap, if householder is disabled (see p. 195);
(viii) hypothermia.

Typical protective measures
Grants and loans to help owner-occupiers and landlords repair or
improve their properties.
Legal powers to control landlords who will not improve environ-
ment.
Provision of new housing of good quality.
Regulations controlling the design of dwellings.

Typical monitoring programme
Studies of samples of housing.
Studies of home accidents.

Principal responsible authorities
Environmental Health Departments of District Councils.
Housing Departments of District Councils and Housing Associa-
tions.
Department of Environment.

Examples of legislative control
Fire Precautions Act (1971).

Domestic appliances

Main health hazards
Burns and scalds.
Electrocution.
Cuts and abrasions.

Typical protective measures
Ergonomically based product design.
Regulations controlling the design and manufacture of domestic appliances.
Information for consumers, such as that given by the British Standards Institute (BSI) 'kitemark'.

Typical monitoring programme
Monitoring of types and causes of home accidents.

Principal responsible authorities
Environmental Health Departments of District Councils.
Manufacturers of domestic appliances.
Department of Prices and Consumer Protection.
European Parliament.

Examples of legislative control
Consumer Safety Act (1978) reinforces the Consumer Safety Act (1961) and a host of other regulations, e.g. the Babies Dummies (Safety) Regulation (1978) and the Electrical Equipment (Safety Amendment) Regulations (1976).

General environment
In addition to the aspects of the environment which directly impinge on an individual there are now important environmental problems which are more difficult to deal with, e.g. noise, dumping of toxic solid waste and radiation. These problems are extremely difficult to control but unless successful measures are adopted the future of life on earth is threatened.

Health monitors

One of the problems in environmental monitoring is that the responsibility is divided among many different authorities and professionals. Four central government departments are involved in the prevention of marine pollution, radiation control and noise other than the Department of Health, which obviously has an interest in health hazards. Closest to the community are the environmental health officers and the community physician. They are the local monitors.

Environmental health officers

Formerly called public health inspector, the environmental health officer is specially trained to monitor the physical environment; an increasing proportion are university graduates. However, he has also to be aware of the social factors which are important because working for a District or City Council brings him into close daily contact with the public and with politicians. Most of his links with central government are with the Department of the Environment and the Department of Health.

Environmental health officers spend most of their time in the prevention of the problems listed in Table 2.1. He can be approached directly by any member of the public or by any professional.

Community physicians

In 1875 an Act of Parliament obliged every local authority to appoint a Medical Officer of Health for the prevention of infectious disease. Over the years the Medical Officer of Health's sphere of responsibility grew. He developed welfare services for the elderly and disabled people and domiciliary nursing and health-visiting services. In 1974 the job of the Medical Officer of Health changed significantly: he lost control of the district nursing and health visiting, as he had lost control of social services 3 years previously; he was transferred from local government to the National Health Service; he was made responsible for coordinating the whole range of health services, including hospital services, and ensuring that they met the needs of the community as effectively and efficiently as possible. His title also

Table 2.1. Preventive approaches of environmental health officers to health problems.

Problem	Preventive approach
Food poisoning	Inspection of food factories, shops and restaurants Education of food-handling staff Investigation of food poisoning cases and outbreaks
Air pollution	Monitoring of air pollution Advice on design of incinerators and chimneys Surveillance of factories and furnaces likely to cause pollution
Injuries and diseases caused by work	Advice to employers and employees on the prevention of occupational diseases and accidents (see p. 165)
Noise	Control of places of entertainment Public education about means of controlling noise
Housing problems	Regular inspection of multioccupied houses Public education

changed. No longer was he a Medical Officer of Health: he became a community physician.

Each District and City Council still has a doctor giving advice on environmental health problems but in many areas this community physician—who is called the 'proper officer' to the Council, or the Medical Officer of Environmental Health—may also be responsible for planning and managing hospital services and so is unable to give the same degree of commitment to the control of infection and the monitoring of the environment as he could formerly. The effects of this trend are, however, mitigated by the increasing skill and expertise of the environmental health officers, who are now much better trained and equipped than were their predecessors, the public health inspectors.

Social environment

It was the changes in the social environment described on p. 6 that brought about changes in the physical environment, thus reducing the mortality from infectious diseases in the nineteenth century. It is the nature of social environment which is the most important influence on the practice of preventive medicine. Information alone is insufficient; consider the lack of action on cigarette smoking when there is adequate information describing the gravity of the problem and the scope for prevention. Social and political changes are necessary before information can be translated into action.

Social changes

Attitudes towards health vary from time to time: attitudes towards the effect that behaviour might have on one's health in the future are different when an individual is fighting a war than when he is living in a time of peace. Similarly, attitudes towards those aspects of life-style that increase the risk of disease alter from time to time. Attitudes to risk factors such as obesity, cigarette smoking, inactivity and drunkenness have changed in the last 20 years and these changes have been beneficial from the perspective of preventive medicine. However, the direction and rate of change has been determined not only by the knowledge that such factors have an influence on health but also by factors that have nothing to do with preventive medicine.

Political changes

The exercise of political power can be a powerful tool for prevention although it can also be an obstacle. The large numbers of laws, regulations, orders and other legal powers that play a part in prevention can be divided into three groups.

Distributive powers

These are perhaps the most important for they are the political changes that alter the distribution of wealth in a society. The changes which took place in nineteenth century Britain redistributed wealth and services, albeit slowly. In more recent times the political changes which stimulated and were implemented by the revolutions in China and Cuba were of fundamental importance in reshaping the distribution of wealth and the pattern of health in these countries. Legislation that improves the opportunities for poor people to use health and social services, e.g. the National Health Service Act of 1946, are also distributive political acts and help to promote prevention.

Regulatory powers

Governments have the power to regulate the actions of individuals and groups of people for the benefit of others or for the benefit of society as a whole. This type of power is used to control employers, house-builders, producers of smoke or chemicals that could pollute water or air, the food industry, and the manufacturers of cars and machines to prevent the types of hazard described in the section on the protection of the physical environment. In general it is unwise to leave preventive medicine to employers, producers or manufacturers. Certainly employers' organizations and industry as a whole have a part to play, but it is usually necessary for the Government to issue a set of regulations which lay down certain minimum safety standards and to specify the sanctions which they will use if these regulations are not obeyed.

Paternalistic powers

The use of political power to control the activities of individuals or groups for the benefit of other people is accepted as appropriate. Politicians may argue about how often governments should use these powers—the early 1980s have seen a campaign against 'too much government' in both Britain and the U.S.A.—but there is general agreement that it is right for a government to use its power in this way. There is, however, much less agreement on the right of government to control an adult whose behaviour is putting only himself at risk.

   Paternalistic powers are more strongly opposed than regulatory powers and the opposition runs right across the political spectrum although the left is, in general, more paternalistic than the right. The types of paternalistic powers that contribute towards the prevention of disease are:

1 Powers that proscribe certain types of behaviour, e.g. driving without a seat belt or riding a motor bike without a crash helmet.

2 Powers that prohibit the sale of certain drugs.

3 Powers that are intended to influence demand, e.g. advertising controls or the use of taxation to increase the price of cigarettes or alcohol.

4 Powers that force preventive services on people such as compulsory vaccination or fluoridation.

It is generally accepted that children need to be protected by such paternalistic powers but there is opposition to their use to control adults. In part, the resistance to paternalistic legislation reflects a mistrust and suspicion of government in general, because paternalistic preventive measures intrude into the pleasures of everyday life in an obvious fashion. Opposition to measures such as seat-belt legislation is therefore a symbol and expression of opposition to other less obvious and less easily comprehended ways in which individual liberty is being eroded by central government. However, it is important to appreciate that many of those who oppose paternalistic powers do so because of a deep concern that the introduction of such measures reduces the liberty and responsibility of the individual and alienates the individual from the government.

Changeurs
Sometimes the introduction of a new law follows a simple course:

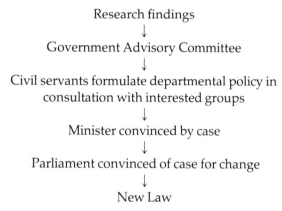

Research findings
↓
Government Advisory Committee
↓
Civil servants formulate departmental policy in
consultation with interested groups
↓
Minister convinced by case
↓
Parliament convinced of case for change
↓
New Law

However, every government department is bombarded with more advice and requests for action than it is possible to handle. Even when the civil servants and the politician who is their master have agreed on a measure they believe to be necessary, the politician first has to find parliamentary time to debate the measure and then has to be able to argue it through. This usually means convincing those politicians who were uncommitted before the issue was introduced to back his proposal, thus allowing him to overcome those who are strongly opposed to his measure. The attitudes which prevail in society—public opinion —influence three stages of this process:

1 the choice of priorities by a Minister and his civil servants;
2 the probability that the Minister will find Parliamentary time to discuss the issue;
3 the attitudes and voting of those politicians who are neither strongly in favour of, or in opposition to, the measure—often the majority of politicians.

Social and political changes are interwoven like warp and weft. Social changes provide the right political climate for a politician to gain sufficient time and attention of parliament to bring about the change he desires. For example, increased public awareness and discussion in the media about lead in petrol resulted in political change in Britain in 1982. Similarly, political change can influence and accelerate changes in public opinion and in the media, e.g. some people cannot believe that cigarettes are as serious a health hazard as the doctors claim because the government allows them to be advertised and sold with so few controls.

Public opinion is, however, a vague and ineffective force for change unless it is harnessed and focussed and, in every case in which the law has been changed, it is possible to identify *changeurs*—individuals or groups whose activities have been of crucial importance in bringing about change.

This all sounds very impressive, big guns banging away at one another with a few charismatic individuals, like Ralph Nader, applying pressure at the right time and in the right place. However, every individual has a part to play and the letters that individuals write to their MP are very important and influential, particularly on the politician who is not strongly committed one way or the other on any particular issue. It is unusual for an MP to receive as many as three letters on a health issue. If he does, and if they are not photocopied or part of an obviously orchestrated lobby, he will take the issue seriously and write to the Minister concerned, who will personally read and answer his, and the constituent's letter. Even if a constituent's letter does not change the way an MP votes, it will influence his attitudes and make him more sympathetic towards the other point of view.

Economics of prevention

Some preventive measures are cheap. The decision to make motor-cyclists wear crash helmets did not cost the State much money but others are expensive and the costs of a number of preventive measures, calculated as cost per life saved, are shown in Table 2.2.

The costs of this type of preventive approach and the implied value of a human life are relatively simple to compute. Often the costs and benefits are more difficult to calculate, particularly where it is not possible to introduce a measure that will deal with every person at risk. More commonly, the objective is to reduce risk not to remove it completely, as in the examples given in Table 2.2; when trying to reduce risks the law of diminishing returns obtains. It can cost as much to reduce the last 10% of risk as it does

Table 2.2. Values of life inferred from several public policy decisions. (After Office of Health Economics (1978) *Renal Failure*, HMSO, London.)

Decision	Implied value of life	Comment and source
Not to introduce child-proof drug containers	£1000 maximum	In 1971 the Government decided not to proceed with the child-proofing of drug containers
Legislation on tractor cabs	£100 000 minimum	In 1969 the fitting of cabs to farm tractors, to reduce mortality risk for drivers, was made compulsory. The cost per annum was estimated at £4000 000 (£40 for each of 100 000 tractors). About 40 lives would be saved yearly
Changes in building regulations as a result of partial collapse of Ronan Point high-rise flats	£20 000 000 minimum or perhaps actual	After a high-rise block of flats partially collapsed, killing some residents, the report of the inquiry recommended changes in the building standards of such blocks. It has been estimated from the change in risk and the costs involved that the implied value of life was £20 000 000
Not to provide treatment for chronic renal failure for a person aged 50	£30 000 (OHE estimate 1976-7 prices)	Particularly in regions where facilities are in short supply, a person over the age of 45 or 50 may stand little chance of being accepted for treatment by dialysis or transplantation

to reduce the first 90% and the cost of abolishing the last per cent may be equal to, or more than, the cost of abolishing the first 99%.

The cost of achieving each percentage reduction in risk and each percentage increase in benefit can be calculated and there comes a point at which one must ask, Is the cost of achieving another per cent of benefit justifiable? or, as an economist would say, At what point does the marginal cost exceed the marginal benefit? It may seem immoral to ask such a question because it is obviously good and justifiable to reduce risk further and to prevent more disease. However, the cost of achieving a further increase in the benefit that the preventive service confers has to be measured not only in terms of money. It is essential to consider the other benefits which that particular amount of money could achieve if differently invested. The economists call this the 'opportunity cost'. Thus, there comes a point at which the opportunity cost of achieving a further increase in benefit is unjustified because of the benefit that will be gained by investing the same amount of resources in another preventive programme.

CHAPTER 3
EDUCATION FOR HEALTH

In the nineteenth century the main causes of disease were environmental. Today the main causes of disease and premature death in developed countries are related to our modern life-style, to factors such as:

1 cigarette smoking;
2 the modern diet;
3 misuse of alcohol and other drugs;
4 the use of motor cars and motor cycles.

Changes in the social environment, such as an increase in the price of cigarettes as a result of government action will, however, not be as effective in reducing the risks of disease as were the measures the government took to change the physical environment in the nineteenth century. Much more responsibility now rests with the individual, and the objective of health education is to help him to make his health choices wisely.

Objectives of health education

At one time the objective of education seemed simple: it was to overcome ignorance, on the assumption that when a person knew about the risks he ran he would change his life-style.

Unfortunately this assumption was wrong. Knowledge alone was not enough to change behaviour. Plenty of people learned about the risks of smoking or of drinking and driving but carried on with these activities: they were better informed but equally at risk. Health educators now appreciate that people are not simply ignorant. On the contrary, the average person has a well-established set of beliefs about health and attitudes towards his health and life-style that are satisfactory for him. The objective of health education is not simply to present facts to fill a void but to present the facts in such a way that a person's beliefs will be changed.

There are four important approaches to health risks depending on the individual's beliefs about:

1 the seriousness of the problem;
2 his own susceptibility;
3 the effectiveness of the action proposed;
4 the cost of taking such action.

Seriousness
Mistaken beliefs: 'Cancer isn't a serious problem these days because of modern methods of treatment.'
'A heart attack is one way to go before you get too old.'
Informed beliefs: 'The results of lung cancer treatment are poor.'
'Heart disease caused by smoking could attack me in my forties.'
Health education message: Lung cancer is incurable but preventable.
Heart attacks are a cause of death and disability in people with young families.

Susceptibility
Mistaken beliefs: 'It won't happen to me.'
'I know someone who had a heart attack and had never smoked.'
Informed belief: 'I am at high risk of heart disease because of my smoking.'
Health education message: Smokers of more than twenty cigarettes a day are three times more likely to experience a heart attack than non-smokers.

Effectiveness
Mistaken belief: 'I've been smoking for years so it's too late for me to stop.'
Informed belief: 'I can reduce the risk I run by stopping smoking.'
Health education message: If you stop smoking your risk of heart disease starts to decline right away and after a couple of years the risk has halved.

Cost
Mistaken belief: 'I'll put on weight and probably start taking valium so I'll finish up worse off.'
Informed belief: 'The net effect on my health is bound to be good;

even if I put on a few pounds that's much less of a risk than smoking.'

Health education message: You can do it; you can stop smoking and you will feel better and fitter as well as reducing your risks of disease.

When speaking to an individual about a health problem, e.g. to a cigarette smoker about heart disease, the simplest way to find out about his beliefs is simply to say, 'I'm not sure how much you know about heart disease. I don't want to bore you if you know a lot about it; could you answer the following questions?

How serious a problem do you think this is among people of your age;
From what you have heard do you think you are particularly at risk, compared with the risk of being killed in a traffic accident for example;
What have you heard about the effects of giving up smoking on your risk of heart disease;
What do you think you would find most difficult or worrying if you gave up smoking?

It should be emphasized that the same approach is equally relevant when speaking to someone with diabetes, epilepsy or any disease that requires medication and is just as important in helping people to take the drugs prescribed for them as in disease prevention.

A change in beliefs does not necessarily lead to a change in attitude or behaviour. In recent years attempts have been made to influence attitudes, using the techniques that some religious cults have used to influence teenagers and that advertisers have developed to change attitudes of consumers, i.e.

$$\text{Change in belief} \rightarrow \text{Change in attitude} \rightarrow \text{Change in behaviour}$$

These changes can be encouraged by education on two fronts, i.e. at school and in the community (see Table 3.1). However, this raises ethical dilemmas. Is it right for health educators to use the same methods as advertisers? Is that education or propaganda?

Table 3.1. Two approaches to influencing social attitudes to smoking as a health risk.

School health education	Public health education
Change in belief	
Basic biological information about heart and lungs	Health warning on cigarette packets
Information about harmful effects of smoking	
Change in attitude	
Use of 'trigger' films and influential pupils to encourage group discussion to change attitudes towards smoking and not smoking	Advertisements stating that those who smoke are less attractive to members of the opposite sex

Health education media

Family

This is the most important influence on health beliefs, attitudes and behaviour.

Within the nuclear family the influence of parents is paramount and when grandparents are near at hand they often exert a continuing influence, notably the influence of the grandmother on childrearing. Education of parents is therefore of prime importance and this is attempted in the following ways.

1 Parentcraft education in secondary schools.

2 Antenatal education.

3 The work of the health visitor with the parents of young children is primarily educational and is conducted both in the home and at child health clinics.

4 The Open University runs a course for parents of young children.

5 Health education of children in schools has an indirect influence on parents.

Friends

In adolescence, friends have a great influence on attitudes and behaviour. Increasingly, therefore, attempts are being made to influence young people's atttitudes so that the individual will find it easier to make decisions reducing the risk of illness. Two examples are:

1 Attempts to help individuals refuse offers of cigarettes by revealing to young people the social pressures on them to conform, the influence of advertising, and suggesting ways in which they can say 'no' without offending their friends.

2 Attempts to change attitudes towards drinking and driving so that the young driver will not be under so much pressure to drink alcohol, and will therefore find it easier not to drink if he is driving.

School
The school is an obvious medium for health education and a number of different approaches are used. These can be grouped under four headings with the following objectives.

Biological: to teach pupils about the human body so that each pupil is well informed about how his or her body functions and what can harm it.

Life skills: to increase pupils' awareness of the social pressures they will face and the resulting influence on their own behaviour.

Decision making: detailed discussions of the decisions each individual has to make concerning, for example, smoking and premarital intercourse, to enable pupils to analyse decisions more logically.

Behavioural modification: the most recent approach, involving group discussions led by the most influential older pupils, who have been appropriately instructed how to influence other young people; the desired objective is a change in behaviour.

The behavioural approach combined with the biological approach is of most interest to the doctor interested in health education, but there is considerable debate about the ethical issues involved: is it education or propaganda?

Organizing health education
In the U.K. control of the curriculum is, with the exception of religious education, the responsibility of the headmaster and board of governors. However, a number of other bodies are involved in the health aspect of education (Fig. 3.1), providing services, materials and general guidelines for the schools activities.

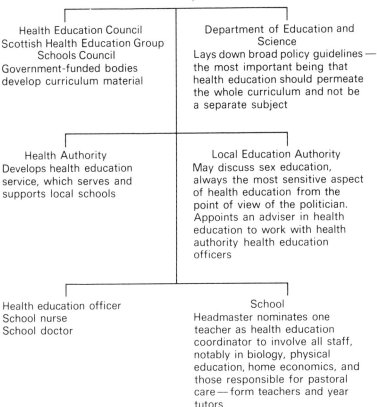

Fig. 3.1. Heirarchy of interacting groups involved in health education as part of the school curriculum.

The media

The main media for public education are:

1 television;
2 newspapers;
3 magazines;
4 advertisements;
5 radio;
6 books.

Each has its own particular contribution to make. Television and advertisements cannot present large amounts of information effectively, but are useful for what is called 'agenda setting', i.e. making people aware that a problem exists.

Television, in addition, is a particularly useful medium for changing attitudes. The other media are also able to influence attitudes but are more suitable media for informing and educating people than for changing behaviour.

Advertising is, of course, not only used to promote health but also the factors associated with ill-health, notably cigarettes and alcohol, e.g. £100 million is spent on the advertising of tobacco in Britain in direct advertising and in the promotion of sporting and artistic events.

The industry's line on advertising is that it is simply concerned with 'brand loyalty', with winning consumers from brand B to brand A, and does not have an effect on the total volume consumed. The effects of a total ban on alcohol advertising in British Columbia in 1972 were insignificant and seem to support this view but there is also evidence to counter it. For example, advertising has played a significant part in the promotion of vodka and although this has been, to a degree, at the expense of whisky there has not been a proportionate fall in the consumption of other spirits; the total volume has in fact increased.

Controls on advertising are, however, important not only because of the effect of advertising on consumption but also because of the effects that controls can have on social attitudes: The advertising of, for example, alcohol makes some young people assume that alcohol consumption is the normal practice for everyone in society. Similarly, many people believe that cigarettes cannot really be as harmful as the doctors say, otherwise the Government would never allow them to be advertised so freely. Advertising controls should, therefore, not only be considered as a means of directly affecting consumption but also as symbols and expressions of society's attitudes.

Controls and checks

In the U.K. the basis of advertising control is the principle of self-regulation.

The Advertising Standards Authority is composed of representatives from both advertising and the media. It issues *The British Code of Advertising Practice*, available from the ASA, 15–17

Ridgemount Street, London WC1E 7AW. Two examples of its controls are reproduced in Fig. 3.2.

The ASA encourages complaints from members of the public who believe that an advertisement is not 'legal, decent, honest and truthful'. Furthermore, the tobacco industry has a 'voluntary agreement' with government which lays down additional rules for sponsorship and advertising.

How well do these controls work? The advertisers think they work very well: many people in preventive medicine also think that they work very well for the industry, but that there is need for the type of government action that has been taken in Norway.

Appendix H   Advertising of cigarettes, of the components of manufactured cigarettes and of hand-rolling tobacco

2.10 Advertisements should not include copy or illustrations which are sexually titillating or which imply a link between smoking and sexual success; nor should any advertisement contain any demonstration of affection in such a way as to suggest romantic or sexual involvement between those portrayed.

2.11 Advertisements should not claim directly or indirectly that it contributes significantly to the attainment of social or business success to smoke, or to smoke a particular brand.

2.12 No advertisement should appear in any publication directed wholly or mainly to young people.

2.13 Advertisements should not feature heroes of the young.

2.14 Advertisements should not imply that smoking is associated with success in sport. They should not depict people participating in any active sporting pursuit or obviously about to do so or just having done so, or spectators at any organized sporting occasion.

Fig. 3.2. Examples of the rules laid down by the Advertising Standards Authority in the *British Code of Advertising Practice, a substitute page for the sixth edition (1983).*

Health educators

Many people are involved in health education but certain professionals have a special interest.

Health education officers

Usually recruited from teaching or nursing, health education officers work for health authorities after special training in health education. There are so few of them—there may only be four for a population of half a million—that their main effort has to be to encourage, persuade, enable and help other professionals, notably teachers and those working in the health service, to become effective health educators. The typical objectives of a health education department are:

1 to encourage every school to nominate one teacher to be health education coordinator and to develop a programme of health education;

2 to help the youth and community service develop in-service training for youth workers and volunteers;

3 to encourage GPs to use the range of materials available for patient education;

4 to help health visitors develop child health clinics as educational centres.

Environmental health officers
Environmental health officers are responsible for:
1 home safety education;
2 education of food-handling staff;
3 education for health and safety at work.

Road-safety education officers
Road-safety education officers are employed by the county engineer's department and are responsible for:
1 road safety education of the public, especially of motorcyclists;
2 road safety education in schools.

Teachers
In primary schools every teacher is involved in some way in health education because of the nature of the primary school curriculum. In secondary schools, two types of teacher will be involved.

1 Those with special skills: e.g. teachers of biology, science, physical education, home economy, civics or social studies.

2 Those with a special relationship with pupils: e.g. form teachers spend 15–30 minutes with their class every day, and may be supported by year tutors in the 'pastoral care' aspect of school life.

The efforts of these groups will be combined by one health education coordinator, appointed by the head teacher (Fig. 3.1). The key to success in secondary education is thus effective co-ordination within the school's curriculum.

Health visitors

All nurses are educators but health visiting is the branch of nursing with a special interest in health education. Health visitors are all State Registered Nurses and qualified midwives who have taken an extra year's training in a university or poly-technic. This training concentrates on human development and psychology and their work is primarily preventive.

Health visitors work with GPs but are not employed by them. Most of their work is with children, with the emphasis on home visiting, although they also organize child health clinics. An increasing proportion of their work is with older people.

Doctors

All doctors are, or should be, educators (*docere*—to teach) but many of them are very ineffective communicators.

GPs have a particular interest in health education and what is called 'patient education', the term used to describe the educa-tion of patients and their relatives about how best to cope with their problems. The GP is in a good position to offer health education because:
1 his opinion on health matters is respected;
2 he has a good relationship with many of the patients on his list—90% of patients come to see him at least once every 5 years.

Health Education Council and Scottish Health Education Group

The Health Education Council is responsible for the development of health education in England, Wales and Northern Ireland, and the Scottish Health Education Group is responsible for Scotland. These two groups are funded by central government and develop health education by:
1 promoting research;
2 using advertising and sponsorship to influence the public;
3 providing training for health educators;
4 developing material that can be used by health educators.

In general, it is best to approach the local health education department before approaching one of these national groups. The local health education department is able to answer most questions.

Self-help groups

Self-care means looking after yourself; self-help means helping other people with the same problem as yourself and therefore yourself also. Self-help groups play a very important part in health education and patient education. Examples of good self-help groups are:

1 Weightwatchers Clubs;
2 Alcoholics Anonymous;
3 CRUSE;
4 The Mastectomy Association;
5 The Colostomy Association.

Does health education work?

Before questioning the effectiveness of health education it is necessary to ask, Are the health educators effective? There is no point in saying a chisel is blunt if the workman is holding the blade and trying to use the handle.

Is the health educator effective?

To be effective the health educator has to have the following five attributes.

Knowledge.

Authority—the health educator has to be respected for his views to be respected.

Trust—if the person trusts and likes the health educator he is more likely to be influenced.

Skill—the average drug representative is better trained at communication than the average doctor; people can be taught to communicate more effectively.

Humility—the ability to accept that the attitudes and opinions of members of the public have to be respected and taken seriously.

Brilliant communicators are probably born and not made, but no matter how good or bad a person is naturally his effectiveness can be improved. He must know the right information and appreciate how to transmit that information effectively. We can at least provide some tips here on how to achieve sympathetic but effective communication.

Always ask the patient's view before starting to give your own.

Look at the person you are speaking to; do not write, look out of the window, fiddle with your pen.

Avoid using too many technical terms but do not be patronizing either.

Let the patient ask questions but, when you encourage a question, pause for at least 30 seconds before assuming that he has no question. Time yourself once or twice; 30 seconds is longer than you think. It seems long to the doctor but it may still be too short for the person to organize his thoughts and ask his question.

Do not try to give too many facts in one interview.

Remember that the written word helps supplement the spoken. Leaflets by themselves are of little use but a well-prepared leaflet can help reinforce the verbal message.

No matter how good you think you are, take a look at yourself with the help of an audio-visual camera.

The effectiveness of health education may be measured with respect to knowledge, attitudes or behaviour. There is evidence that all three can be influenced but, without increased investments in health education, it would be unrealistic to expect that health education alone can have a significant impact on the incidence of preventable disease.

CHAPTER 4
PREVENTIVE HEALTH SERVICES

In the nineteenth century, prevention was achieved primarily by environmental engineering, through the development of public health services. During the twentieth century there has been the development of personal health services—personal preventive health services and treatment services.

The traditional way of classifying this type of preventive health service is to group the services according to the stage of the disease at which they are intended to have their effect (Table 4.1).

Table 4.1. Primary, secondary and tertiary prevention.

Natural history of disease	Preventive measure	Example
Person at risk of disease	Primary prevention	Advice on obesity given to middle-aged men to reduce risk of maturity-onset of diabetes
Person has disease but is unaware of it because it is not yet causing symptoms	Secondary prevention: this is often associated with the term 'screening'	Testing for glucose in the urine of a middle-aged, obese man who has no symptoms and feels well
Person has symptomatic disease	Tertiary prevention: this is simply another term for clinical medicine in which the aims are prevention of compli-cations and premature death	Careful surveillance of a person on oral hypo-glycaemic drugs

This approach has an attractive simplicity but it also has its drawbacks. One obvious disadvantage is that it is often difficult to determine when a person has begun to develop a disease. For example, can giving advice to stop smoking and lose weight to an asymptomatic 35-year-old man really be regarded as primary prevention when it is almost certain he already has atherosclerosis? Because of this problem some people started to talk about 'prevention in the asymptomatic phase', grouping together primary and secondary prevention, but this is not completely satisfactory and we shall therefore use the traditional terms 'primary', 'secondary' and 'tertiary' prevention in this chapter.

Primary preventive services

The objective in primary prevention is to prevent the disease process from starting. Examples of services for primary prevention are:

1 health education (see Chapter 3);
2 immunization;
3 provision of vitamin supplements to babies;
4 fluoridation;
5 meals on wheels for older people.

Immunization and fluoridation are in a different class from health education. The link between the input and the outcome, i.e. between the provision of the service and the prevention of disease, is not so direct in health education, whereas in fluoridation and immunization the link is simple and direct:

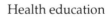

Fluoridation of water supplies → Increase in blood fluoride levels → Reduction of incidence of caries

With health education the chain is longer and other influences also play their part:

Health education
↓
Interaction with indiviudal's own beliefs and attitudes
↓
Change of belief and attitudes
↓
Interaction with other influences such as friends and the media
↓
Intention to change behaviour
↓
Behaviour change

Other measures could be taken that would affect the primary prevention of disease, but these are not usually classified as preventive health services because the relationship between the introduction of the measure and the prevention of disease is even longer and more complicated than that illustrated for the effect of health education. These preventive services are those measures which would:

1 prevent poverty;
2 provide every family with satisfactory housing;
3 ensure equal access to health services of good quality for all people;
4 provide jobs for everyone.

There seems little doubt that such measures would, in the long term, lead to the prevention of disease. However, there is considerable uncertainty about the manner in which being a member of a 'lower social class' has an adverse influence on health, and there is no simple link between the provision of better housing or full employment and the prevention of disease. It therefore seems more appropriate to consider political measures rather than personal preventive health services, although the prevention of poverty and the narrowing of the gap between the social classes would lead to the prevention of disease.

Secondary preventive services

In many diseases there comes a stage at which the disease is untreatable and, unless the doctor sees the sufferer before that stage is reached he cannot treat the disease effectively. The referral of problems before they reach this late, untreatable stage by the patient himself and by his GP is, therefore, very important. It is a simple step from this observation to propose that the earlier treatment is started the better; that it would be still more effective to start treating diseases before they had even reached the symptomatic stage, which is only the tip of the iceberg of disease (Fig. 4.1). To do this, of course, requires the doctor (i) to initiate contact with those who are known to be at risk of a particular disease and (ii) to offer them the diagnostic tests which would reveal whether or not they have a disease in the early symptomatic form.

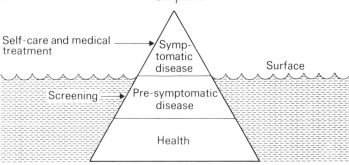

Fig. 4.1. The iceberg of disease.

The decade of expansion

This is the *rationale* behind screening; and the argument seemed so sensible in the 1960s that considerable enthusiasm was generated and a number of screening services were introduced on an experimental basis (Table 4.2).

Table 4.2. Examples of screening services introduced in the 1960s.

Disease screened for	Test
Cancer of the rectum and sigmoid colon	Annual sigmoidoscopy
Coronary heart disease	Annual electrocardiography
Glaucoma	Regular aplanation tonometry for older people
Anaemia	Regular haemoglobin estimations

Often a number of screening tests were given at the same time in what was called 'multiphasic screening' where the objective was not only to discover asymptomatic disease but to find symptomatic disease that had not been recognized by the person being screened. Of course, this was not a new concept. Infant welfare and school health clinics had had screening programmes for 70 years concerned not only with primary prevention but with the early detection of disease. But the application of this principle to adults did not develop until the 1950s and only flourished in the 1960s.

The decade of reappraisal

In the 1970s, however, the tide started to turn as people became concerned about certain aspects of screening.

Let us take the example of a woman who notices a breast lump and who is naturally anxious. She will seek help and readily agree to a biopsy, accepting that the operation carries some risk, that doctors are not completely infallible and can only try to do their best and that she will have a small scar on her breast. This is the traditional contract between doctor and patient. The position of a woman found to have a lump in a breast cancer screening programme is different. She is made anxious by the doctor, she is exposed to the risk of a general anaesthetic and operation by the doctor and she will have a scar because of the doctor's actions. If, at the end of all this, the lump is proved to be cancerous this anxiety and disturbance will be justified, provided that the doctor is sure that the early detection of breast cancer improves the chance of cure and survival, something that is not yet certain (see p. 180). If, on the other hand, the lump is benign the woman's anxiety and suffering are even more difficult to justify. She has suffered because she might have had cancer, but did not, and perhaps the best way to justify her suffering is to say that if some women are to be cured of cancer others have to suffer. Now this is an issue for public debate but it is obvious that the contract between doctor and the person being screened is completely different from the traditional doctor–patient relationship. The 'costs' to the patient of screening may therefore be:

1 inconvenience;
2 anxiety;
3 discomfort;
4 risk that the screening procedure may be harmful;
5 risk of being labelled as 'sick' or 'at risk'.

The potential benefit must outweigh these costs and even more rigorous criteria of safety and efficiency must be satisfied for screening than for new therapies.

The evaluation of screening tests

Criteria for the evaulation of screening programmes have been listed as follows.

1 The condition screened for should be an important one.

2 There should be an acceptable treatment for patients with the disease.

3 The facilities for diagnosis and treatment should be available.

4 There should be a recognized latent or early symptomatic stage.

5 There should be a suitable test or examination which should neither miss many cases of the disease, i.e. give false negative results, nor diagnose disease when the person is healthy, i.e. give false positive results. The test must be sensitive and specific.

SeNsitive tests give few false Negatives;
sPecific tests give few false Positives.

---

6 The test or examination should be acceptable to the population.

7 The natural history of the condition, including the development from a latent to a declared disease, should be adequately understood.

8 There should be an agreed policy on whom to treat as patients.

9 The cost of screening (including diagnosis and subsequent treatment of patients) should be economically balanced in relation to expenditure on medical care as a whole.

10 Screening should be a continual process and not a 'one off' project.

Economic considerations

Because resources are always limited, the cost–benefit balance of any screening procedure is an important consideration. The inevitable delay, which may be prolonged, between screening and the realization of any potential benefit makes assessment of the value especially difficult. Moreover, because of the large numbers likely to be involved in any screening procedure, financial considerations loom large.

Even if a screening procedure can be shown to be effective as a preventive measure, its feasibility may be excluded by its cost. Because the demand for medical care always exceeds the resources available, the question of priorities is ever present. Economic evaluation of screening is further hindered by the difficulties in measuring both cost and benefit. Apart from the cost of the screening procedure itself, there are indirect ones such as the cost of attending the screening venue and of time lost from work. The benefits in economic terms are even more difficult to evaluate but this problem is not, of course, peculiar to screening. The measurement of economic gain from any medical intervention is rarely simple and the remoteness of the possible benefit from the screening aggravates this problem.

The current position
The annual 'check-up' is now considered to be ineffective by most people interested in preventive medicine and the only screening procedures recommended for healthy adults in Britain are:
1 cervical cytology;
2 measurement of high blood pressure;
3 regular dental examinations.
    Regular dental examinations are performed by the dental surgeon and the other two tests by doctors or nurses. The trend is for these tests to be carried out in general practice, not through a distinct screening programme but as an integral part of the general medical services offered by the GP to his patient.
    More than 90% of people visit the GP at least once in every 5 years for the relief of some symptom or to discuss a problem with him. If the opportunity is taken to offer the person blood-pressure measurement and cervical cytology at one of these visits then 90% of the population can be covered without having to write letters to people or carry out screening 'campaigns'. This is known as an opportunistic approach to prevention, and is part of a trend in general practice to make full use of the opportunity offered by these visits to the doctor.
    However, for this to be an effective way of detecting disease early it is necessary for the GP, with the help of the practice nurse, to (i) make good use of the appointments made by the patients; and (ii) have a record system that will allow him to identify which of his patients have not been seen at the end of the 5 year period. If he has both the right approach and the right record system he will be able to detect disease early and to practice effective preventive medicine.

Tertiary preventive services

Tertiary prevention is more than the effective treatment of established disease. It implies:

1 anticipation of problems that might arise and sensitivity to related medical, or social, problems;

2 organization of health services so that people who are suffering from a chronic disease are kept under surveillance.

This type of approach, which can be practised in either general practice or the hospital, is now called anticipatory care. Good anticipatory care is demonstrated in the following examples.

Enquiring about the health of the wife looking after a husband severely disabled by Parkinson's disease when she presents at the surgery to collect a repeat prescription for him.

Taking the blood pressure of a man who consults because he wishes relief for backache.

Arranging for a cervical smear test for a woman who has brought her child to the health centre and who has not had a smear test for 5 years.

Excluding the possibility that a person whose blood pressure is raised also has diabetes.

Having a register in which all patients with high blood pressure in a practice are recorded, and which can reveal those patients who have not kept appointments.

Counselling the teenage children of someone who has had a stroke.

Having a record system which allows the GP to detect which of his 80-year-old patients have not made contact with the practice in the previous year.

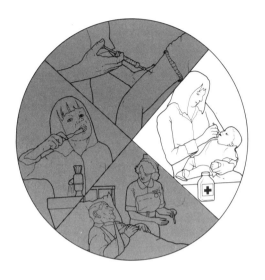

CHAPTER 5
PREVENTION IN CHILDHOOD

In childhood, as at other ages, there is a marked difference in health in different social classes. This was identified in the Royal College of General Practitioners Report on *Healthier Children. Thinking Prevention* (1970) which found that:
1 the infant mortality rate in social class V (the poorest class) is 2.5 times the rate in social class I;
2 mortality rates from accidents are five times as high in poorer social classes than in richer;
3 traffic and home accidents are more common in poorer social classes.

The relationship between social class and health is complex and poorly understood but the following factors appear to be important.
1 Poor housing conditions.
2 Poverty.
3 Unsatisfactory physical environment, e.g. lack of safely accessible play space.
4 Less use of health services, e.g. vaccination, by those more in need.
These are practical factors but there are undoubtedly other cultural or social factors which have an influence.
1 The feeling of powerlessness resulting from prolonged unemployment.
2 The feeling of worthlessness resulting from rejection by employers and lack of the amenities and possessions which are regarded as 'normal' by society, e.g. a house.
3 The feeling that only the here and now is of importance, resulting from years, and sometimes generations, of a life-style dominated by insecurity in which house and job could be lost without notice, and in which savings, mortgages and future planning were never possible.

This is not to argue that there is a 'cycle of deprivation' that cannot be influenced, only to emphasize the importance of social and economic factors in the promotion of child health. In addition to the specific measures suggested in this chapter there is therefore a need to introduce policies which improve housing, improve education, and prevent poverty. Such changes would not, of course, immediately abolish social-class differences in health in childhood but without such changes specific preventive measures will only have a limited effect and the health gap between rich and poor will persist.

Preventive steps to better health

The easiest way to consider prevention in childhood is to consider the different stages of the life of a child. However, the different types of preventive service do not simply follow one another. Their effects are cumulative because the more successful prevention is at one stage the more likely will be the success of preventive efforts in subsequent stages, e.g. the child born healthy because of good antenatal care will benefit to a greater degree from the preventive measures in infancy.

Specific services—preconception

Prevention in childhood starts before conception. Two services are of particular importance—family planning and genetic counselling (Table 5.2).

Specific services—*in utero*

Once the child has been conceived a new set of preventive measures becomes relevant. These may be divided into two types—educational and medical.

Education in pregnancy

Public education
Preparation for parenthood starts in childhood with the lessons a pregnant woman and her husband have learned from their own upbringing. This is supplemented by parentcraft education in

Table 5.1. Preconception preventive services.

Service	Benefit	Obstacles
Family planning	Of particular importance to very young women	Low uptake of service by those most at risk
	Of importance to women near the menopause	
	Important to mentally handicapped people	
Genetic counselling service	For older women because the risk of Down's syndrome rises with age	Lack of skilled genetic counsellors
	For those who have had one handicapped child or who have a family history of a disease that is genetically determined	Failure of professionals to refer people at risk to available counselling services

schools although this is by no means universal, boys and more able children being less likely to receive this type of health education. In pregnancy, antenatal health education is offered by community midwives and health visitors, by voluntary organizations such as the National Childbirth Trust, and by books and magazines produced by commercial publishers and by the Health Education Council. The objectives of antenatal education are listed below.

To prepare parents for the changes that the baby will bring.
To teach the basic principles of child care.
To dispel the fear of labour.
To encourage healthy habits in pregnancy, e.g. smoking cessation, exercise and a prudent diet.
To encourage attendance at antenatal clinics and complement the education given at clinic visits.

Professional education

This is equally important. Professionals must be given the right type of education. Not only should they know how to deliver preventive services effectively, they should also appreciate the emotional aspects of pregnancy and the right of each woman to be treated with understanding. The objectives of professional education are summarized below.

To teach professionals the skills needed to detect abnormalities in pregnancy.

To educate professionals about the beliefs and attitudes of pregnant women and their husbands.

To encourage the development of services that are sensitive to individual need as well as being effective in covering the whole population at risk.

Preventive services

Early and regular attendance at antenatal clinics is important. It allows the early detection of maternal diseases that can harm the fetus—notably pre-eclampsia, hypertension, diabetes and anaemia—and the early detection of fetal disease, thus allowing the pregnant woman and her husband the option of a termination.

Because the 'preventive measure' is usually termination of pregnancy this aspect of preventive medicine bristles with ethical problems and the education of pregnant women should cover not only the changes occurring within them but also the tests being performed on them, their implications and significance (Table 5.2).

Specific measures in labour

Much has been made of the difference between 'natural childbirth' and 'high technology obstetrics' but there is a continuum between the two. Two principles of prevention in labour are particularly important.

Table 5.2. Common tests performed antenatally for diagnosing congenital abnormalities. (After Macfarlane, J. A. (1980) *Child Health Pocket Consultant*. Grant McIntyre, London.)

Abnormality	Test	Optimal timing of test
Anencephaly and spina bifida	Alpha fetoprotein level in blood, followed if necessary by an amniocentesis*	14–18 weeks after conception 14–18 weeks after conception
Congential rubella	Blood test for antibodies	If contact or disease suspected, separated tests to show rise in antibody levels
Down's syndrome (in mothers aged over 35–40 years)	Amniocentesis*	14–18 weeks after conception
Rhesus isoimmunization	Blood tests	At regular intervals during pregnancy if suspected
Sex-linked inherited diseases (where specific indications)	Amniocentesis*	14–18 weeks after conception
Syphilis	Routine blood test	At booking
Toxoplasmosis	Blood test for antibodies (in endemic areas only)	At booking, and later to check rising antibody levels

*Amniocentesis is a complicated procedure which causes spontaneous abortion in about 1 in 100, and therefore is only carried out when there are specific indications.

1 The degree of supervision and intervention should be appropriate to the degree of risk; some fetuses are much more at risk than others.

2 The degree of sensitivity and respect towards the wishes of the pregnant woman and her husband should be equally high whatever the degree of intervention—the use of 'high technology' need not, and should not, reduce the woman's enjoyment of the birth of her child.

Thus, there needs to be a range of obstetric services from delivery at home to the specialist obstetric centre.

Home		GP		Consultant unit in		Regional
delivery	→	unit	→	district general hospital	→	specialist unit

Women in pregnancy should be guided to the appropriate unit before the start of labour and transferred from one to another should the need arise during labour.

Specific measures in infancy

In the first month of life
In the first month of life the hazards are high, but at no time is the relationship between prevention in one stage of life and prevention in the next more obvious. If the preventive measures during pregnancy have been effective the risks in the early days of life are minimized, because the most important cause of death and handicap is low birth weight and its associated complications; other common causes are congenital abnormalities and infections.

In the early days of life, screening is carried out for two disorders—phenylketonuria and congenital hypothyroidism.

The community midwife is the key worker in the first 2 weeks of life. However, at 14 days she hands over to the health visitor who coordinates prevention in infancy.

Prevention in infancy
Prevention in infancy has four main interrelated themes. These are illustrated in Fig. 5.1.

Education
This is the most important preventive measure. Without it the other objectives cannot be attained. There are two important sources of education: the informal, e.g. parents, grandparents, sisters-in-law, friends, women's magazines and books; and formal, of which the most important is the health visitor who educates both during home visits and child health clinics.

Nutrition
There are two interrelated objectives of nutrition—the mainten-

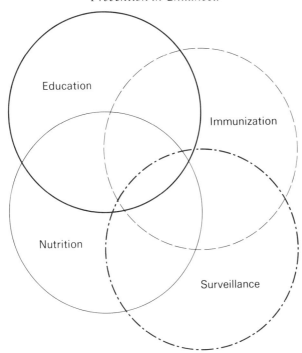

Fig. 5.1. Venn diagram of the four main interrelated themes of prevention in infancy.

ance of breast-feeding for as long as possible and the prevention of obesity.

Immunization
The immunization schedule for the first year of life is shown in Table 5.3. In recent years the proportion of infants immunized has fallen and this has been due principally to fears about whooping-cough vaccine. The reluctance of parents to expose their child to any risk is understandable and the prominence given to the risks in the press has led to an increase in the refusals of offers of immunization.

Surveillance
The surveillance of these three themes and of the child's development is orchestrated by the health visitor in an integrated pro-

Table 5.3. Suggested schedule for immunization of babies (based on DHSS recommendations). After Macfarlane, J. A. (1980) *Child Health Pocket Consultant*. (Grant McIntyre, London.)

Age	Vaccine	Dose
3 months	Diphtheria Tetanus Pertussis	0.5 ml of combined vaccine by intramuscular injection
	Polio	3 drops orally
5 months	Diphtheria Tetanus Pertussis	0.5 ml of combined vaccine by intramuscular injection
	Polio	3 drops orally
9 months	Diphtheria Tetanus Pertussis	0.5 ml of combined vaccine by intramuscular injection
	Polio	3 drops orally
12–24 months	Measles	0.5 ml reconstituted vaccine by intramuscular injection or by subcutaneous injection

gramme of visits to the child's own home and to the child health clinic. Despite all these measures, however, many children still die as cot deaths.

The mystery of cot deaths
More than one-half of children dying between 1 week and 1 year of age die unexpectedly at home. The cause of cot deaths is unknown so that there are no specific preventive measures. The principal approaches therefore are research and support for bereaved parents who are distraught with grief and guilt.

Specific measures in childhood

The commonest cause of death in childhood is the accident—home accidents in young children, with road accidents becoming more common as children grow older. The most common causes of death in these two age groups are:

1–4 years —1 Accidents
           2 Congenital abnormalities
           3 Pneumonia and respiratory disease
5–14 years—1 Accidents
           2 Cancer
           3 Congenital abnormalities

Accident prevention

The same principles of prevention apply for all types of accident. First the cause has to be determined and then the three preventive steps illustrated in Fig. 5.2 can be taken.

Child education

Road-safety education is the responsibility of the highways authorities and county and city councils; road-safety training officers are employed in these departments.

Home-safety education is the responsibility of health visitors and environmental health officers.

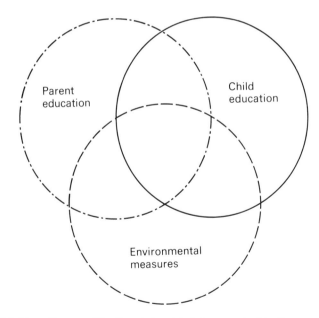

Fig. 5.2. Venn diagram of the three interrelated steps required for the prevention of accidents in childhood.

Parental education

Parents need to be taught not only about the environmental hazards their children face but also, and equally important, about the difficulties that children have in learning about risks and dangers. In many accidents the principal reason is that the parent has expected too much of the child, e.g. expecting a 4-year-old child to cross busy roads alone.

Environmental measures

The design of houses, flats, playgrounds, roads, toys and household appliances are factors in accident causation and prevention. Sometimes manufacturers make changes of their own volition. On other occasions legislative changes are required to ensure that a product conforms to safety regulations (see p. 23). The EEC Consumer Protection Act and similar measures introduced in our own Parliament ensure that manufacturers see that it is in their own interests to think of the safety of their products.

Immunization

The child's immune defences are further strengthened throughout childhood. The suggested schedule of immunization is given in Table 5.4

Table 5.4. Suggested schedule for immunization of children (based on DHSS recommendations). After Macfarlane, J. A. (1980) *Child Health Pocket Consultant.* (Grant McIntyre, London.)

Age	Vaccine	Dose
4½–5½ years	Diphtheria Tetanus Polio	0.5 ml of combined vaccine by intra-muscular injection 3 drops orally
10–15 years (No longer universal in UK)	BCG	0.1 ml by intradermal injection (tuberculin-negative children only) Multidose guns as an alternative
11–13 years (girls only)	Rubella	0.5 ml reconstituted vaccine by subcutaneous injection *only*. (Should be given to all girls whether or not they have had rubella)
15–18 years	Tetanus Polio	0.5 ml given by intra-muscular injection 3 drops orally

The School Health Service

The School Health Service was introduced in 1907 (see p. 8). In the first decades of its work it was primarily concerned with the detection and treatment of physical disease. The position has changed now and school doctors and school nurses are now principally involved in four areas of work.

1 Immunization.

2 Routine screening of all school entrants.

3 Children with emotional and behavioural problems; working with social workers and educational social workers, who are concerned primarily with children who are absent excessively, and colleagues in child psychiatry and child-guidance services.

4 Handicapped children, who are increasingly being educated in ordinary schools.

Health education

This is a vitally important health service preparing the children for the next stage of life—adolescence.

In spite of the development of all these services, many children still suffer at home from ill-treatment by their parents.

The mystery of child abuse

Child abuse has no single cause. A number of contributory factors have been identified but these are not so specific that a preventive programme can be worked out. Emphasis must therefore be placed on the preventive approach.

Early detection of children at risk.

Careful surveillance.

Good cooperation between all the agencies involved.

CHAPTER 6
PREVENTION IN ADOLESCENCE

The health problems of people in adolescence receive little attention because the mortality rates are low and because young people make relatively little use of the health service.

The pattern of health

Mortality in adolescence
In the U.K. the common causes of death are road-traffic accidents and cancer. The cancers that occur in adolescence are not preventable but a proportion of the road-traffic accidents are. Table 6.1 lists the three types of road-traffic accidents in adolescence, and the means of prevention. However, the relative ineffectiveness of these approaches can only be appreciated when the beliefs and attitudes of young people are taken into account and these will be discussed in the next section of this chapter.

Prevention of homicide and violent behaviour
In some American cities homicide is the most common cause of death in young males, and in many countries violence is a common cause of hospital admission. This is obviously a social problem but, since violence has important medical consequences, the United States Surgeon General includes homicide in his review of the scope for preventing the United States' main health problems. Because the causes of violence are social there are few simple preventive measures which will reduce the prevalence of football hooliganism or the incidence of homicide. There are, however, two measures which could help. One is the introduction of measures to prevent the consumption of alcohol at, and preferably before, football matches, for much of the violence is probably precipitated by alcohol. The other measure which is of relevance in the U.S. is an amendment in the gun laws to make the possession and distribution of firearms, and therefore their use, much more difficult.

Table 6.1. Types of road-traffic accident in adolescence and their means of prevention.

Nature of problem	Means of prevention
Cycle	
These occur in the younger end of the age range. They are rarely caused by mechanical failure of brakes although many bikes are in poor repair. Most commonly they are caused by mistakes made by either the cyclist, particularly when turning to the right, or by drivers	Separation of cycles from traffic by means of cycle tracks Education of cyclists about risks of cycling
Motorcycle	
These occur more commonly among inexperienced riders and those riding more powerful bikes. It is important to emphasize that in many accidents the motor cyclist is not to blame	Introduction of a more difficult test for motor cyclists Development of motor-cyclist training schemes Introduction of rules to restrict the use of more powerful bikes to older motor cyclists Compulsory wearing of crash helmets
Car	
These occur among an older age group and in the majority of accidents alcohol is an important cause	General measures taken to try to prevent drinking and driving Particular educational measures aimed at young people with the objective of persuading young people that it is socially unacceptable for the person who is driving to be pushed to drink alcohol

Such measures, however, though simple to describe are difficult to implement, for they impinge upon certain actions that are regarded by some people as inviolable; namely, the right to consume alcohol at a football match in the U.K. or to carry a gun in the U.S.

Disability in adolescence

The main scope for the prevention of disability is the prevention of road traffic accidents, some of which result in permanent disabilities, e.g. paraplegia or brain damage. Other common causes of disability in adolescence are disorders which developed before, or around, the time of birth, e.g. spina bifida or cerebral palsy.

Use of hospital services
Official statistics often make it difficult to determine the use of health services by adolescents because they are often grouped in the age groups 5–14 and 15–34 years. If, however, the statistics for people in their teens are grouped together certain preventable problems can be identified. These and their means of prevention are described in Table 6.2.

However any programme for prevention, whether it is going to depend principally on legislation, or education or a combination of both, requires the beliefs and attitudes of young people to be taken into account.

Health beliefs and attitudes

In this context, there is insufficient space to review all the beliefs and attitudes that are experienced during adolescence. Only those which have a direct relevance to preventive medicine will be discussed.

Health beliefs
In Chapter 4, four types of health belief were discussed, i.e. beliefs about seriousness, susceptibility, the benefit of taking preventive action, and the costs of taking preventive action. We will now examine these in greater detail.

Beliefs about seriousness
Adolescents who have never known the effects of serious illness may not be worried by talk of 'accidents' or 'serious disease'. To them the result of an accident may be seen as no more than a plaster on a broken arm which makes a child the centre of attraction. Accidents and illness are seen as rewarding situations, with extra sympathy and attention and time off school as the rewards, rather than situations they should strive to avoid.

Beliefs about susceptibility
Many children perceive themselves to be invulnerable: in part

Table 6.2. Preventable problems in adolescence.

Nature of problem	Means of prevention
Trauma Two types of injury dominate the picture: 1 Minor head injuries which are responsible for a large number of admissions, each of short duration. These result from sport, fighting and road-traffic accidents 2 Serious injuries caused by road-traffic accidents, e.g. fractured shaft of femur. These are less common than head injuries but require a longer period of hospitalization.	Prevention of road-traffic accidents
Pregnancy May result in: 1 Abortion which may be done in a day unit 2 Delivery which requires hospitalization	Prevention of pregnancy is very difficult. Education may be ineffective and where girls under 16 are concerned it is the cause of ethical and political debate, with many people convinced of the fact that education about sex promotes and encourages promiscuity. There is no evidence that this is the case. There is neither the evidence, however, to prove that ignorance is a major cause of teenage pregnancy. Many girls who become pregnant know the 'facts of life'. Provision of a young person's family planning clinic in which staff are skilled and sensitive and which is easily accessible plays an important part in preventing pregnancy
Overdose Although it is impossible to classify all suicide attempts as being either self-destructive or manipulative, those that occur in adolescence tend to be motivated more by an attempt to influence other people, e.g. to make them feel guilty or sympathetic	This is difficult because the taking of an overdose is the result of so many social and cultural influences, but the provision of counselling services for distressed young people probably has a part to play in helping them cope with crises without using an overdose

because they have only intimations of mortality and in part because the adolescent who is so uncertain of his social position and identity may cope with this uncertainty by presenting a very confident face to the world.

Beliefs about benefits
The young person advised to behave in a certain way may not believe that a change in behaviour will have any effect. He may believe that cigarettes do not cause harm because he knows old men, or even one old man, who has smoked for years, or he may not believe that motor-cycle training will be beneficial because he does not know anyone who has been killed in a road traffic accident, even though none of his friends have had training.

Beliefs about the costs of preventive action
The adolescent may believe that the costs of preventive action will be prohibitively high, e.g. a 14-year-old boy may believe that if he refuses the offer of a cigarette he will be reviled and expelled from his group, or a 15-year-old girl may believe that her boy-friend will not love her if she refuses to have sexual intercourse with him. Adolescents almost always overestimate the social costs of refusing to conform but that is a very difficult belief to change.

Attitudes to health (Table 6.3)

Attitudes to old age
To the person aged 15 the rewards of prevention, namely survival, are unattractive. Few young people are excited by the prospects of survival into middle or old age—to some even the age of 24 seems 'old'—and death therefore may hold no fears. To such young people there is little attraction in adopting the changes suggested by health educators.

Attitudes to the future
Although some young people have a clear view of the future and modify their behaviour to achieve a long-term goal, e.g. by studying every evening and at weekends to achieve a place in medical school, many live in the present. The promise of benefits

Table 6.3. Health beliefs in adolescence.

Beliefs and attitudes; obstacles to prevention	Implications for education
Old age	Avoid references to the prevention of death in middle age; it is not an argument that cuts any ice with young people
	Concentrate on the prevention of disability rather than the prevention of death; some youngsters are impressed by the fact that motor-cycle accidents cause not only death but also paraplegia
The future	Focus on the short-term benefits that result from taking exercise or stopping smoking, i.e. emphasis should be given to the effect on the way the individual feels and looks rather than to the reduction of risk
Authority Adolescence is a time in which authority is challenged as the child establishes his or her own set of attitudes and values in a dialectic with parents, teachers and health educators. Health warnings such as 'don't start smoking' may therefore be challenged and ignored simply because they offer an opportunity for young people to reject attempts by authority to influence their beliefs and attitudes	Avoid an authoritarian approach. Wherever possible young people should be helped to debate issues among themselves. They need information on which to base their discussion and may stimulate or even provoke the discussion, but attempts to impose values or influence attitudes will be resisted
Adult behaviour Paradoxically, the adolescent who resists and rejects adult attitudes and values may be attracted by adult behaviour, or what he considers to be the behaviour of the mature adult, e.g. smoking, drinking alcohol and sexual intercourse are seen as 'grown-up' behaviour by many young people who partake in these activities, while rejecting the attempts of adults to dissuade them from smoking, drinking and sexual intercourse because they wish to challenge authority	Attempts have to be made to present young people with an alternative image of the adult, grown-up world, e.g. by identifying attractive adults who do not smoke or drink heavily
	Young people should be taught the techniques of advertising and shown how advertisers are trying to influence their behaviour, e.g. by the sponsorship of sport by cigarette companies

Table 6.3. Continued

Beliefs and attitudes; obstacles to prevention	Implications for education
Behaviour of peers	
Because the adolescent is in a state of existential uncertainty during the transition from the child who shares his parents' values and attitudes to the adult who has his own set of attitudes and values, he needs the support of his peers more than the child needs support from other children. The values, attitudes and therefore behaviour of the other members of the group influence the individual. If they all smoke he may smoke simply so that he is not different	Education of the individual has to be complemented by education of the group One of the objectives of health education should be to let the adolescent appreciate the social pressures he has to cope with; not only the pressure of advertising but also the pressure imposed by his friends In some schools, particularly in the U.S.A., the young person is given instruction specifically on how to resist social pressure
Risk and danger	
To the typical health educator, doctor, nurse, or teacher, with a house and a mortgage and family responsibilities, risks and dangers are situations to be avoided. Adolescents, however, may have a different view, particularly those adolescents who do not experience the excitement created by examinations or sport. They may not try to avoid risks pointed out to them, in fact they may be attracted to them	Advice on risks should be given in a neutral tone, avoiding heavily charged warnings against 'risks' or 'dangers', e.g., instead of trying to influence young motor-cyclists to be 'safe' riders, encouragement should be given to them to become 'good' riders. Safety has such a boring image that any advice linked to safer riding may be rejected whereas the same advice linked to 'better' or 'more skilful' riding may be accepted

in the future to a group of young people who are unemployed and who see no hope of employment is of little relevance.

Attitudes to authority
Health education is often perceived as emanating from 'authority' by young people, and as part of a healthy adolescence is opposition to authority the health education messages may be rejected.

Attitudes to adult behaviour
The attitudes of young people to the behaviour of older people is

apparently inconsistent because they are keen to adopt certain types of behaviour—notably cigarette smoking, and the consumption of alcohol—while refusing to adopt certain other types of behaviour, for example careful road use. However, there is a consistent pattern because young people adopt the behaviour of the type of adult they would like to appear to be and, for many young people, the image of the sophisticated, self-assured adult is associated with cigarette-smoking, alcohol-consumption and promiscuity.

Attitudes to risk

To many doctors and teachers risks should be avoided wherever possible. To many young people, on the other hand, risks are less frightening; indeed they may be attractive, in part because authority advocates risk avoidance as 'good behaviour', in part because of the excitement they offer. The enjoyment of excitement in adolescence should not be underestimated. Young people enjoy excitement and it is pointless simply to repeat the word 'don't' to them. Young people need excitement and challenges and if life offers neither employment nor an exciting environment the argument that they should not smoke because it is safer is not likely to have much impact.

CHAPTER 7
PREVENTION IN ADULT LIFE

Scope for prevention

Causes of mortality
In the U.K., as in all developed countries, the causes of death in adult life are relatively few in number. Circulatory disease, including heart attacks and strokes, cancers, respiratory diseases, and accidents account for the great majority of adult deaths. Accidents, particularly road traffic accidents, are relatively more common in the early years of adult life, becoming relatively less important as the numbers dying from accidents decrease and the numbers dying from the other three causes increase (Fig. 7.1).

Causes of disability and handicap
Rheumatoid arthritis.
Ischaemic heart disease.
Chronic bronchitis.
Stroke.
Multiple sclerosis.
Accidents.
Emotional problems—anxiety and depression.
Alcohol abuse.

The scope for prevention of both premature death and disability is considerable if mortality rates for people aged between 25 and 64 years in the U.K. are expressed as a percentage of the lowest mortality rate observed in Sweden, the U.S.A., Canada and the U.K. (Fig. 7.2). The proportion of mortality that is preventable can be calculated.

Mortality in this age group in the U.K. is on average 50% above the lowest observed mortality which is, of course, not the

74

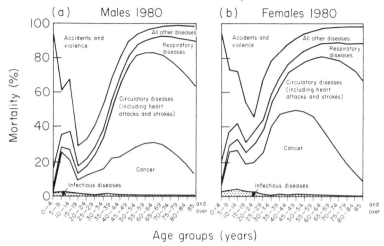

Fig. 7.1. Causes of death in adult life for males and females during 1980. Source: Office of Population Censuses and Surveys, General Register Office (Scotland), and General Register Office (N. Ireland).

lowest possible mortality. In addition, six of the eight major causes of disability are, in part, preventable and certain risk factors can be identified that offer scope for prevention.

Risk factors in adult life

1 Cigarette smoking.
2 Obesity.
3 Substance abuse, including the abuse of prescribed medication.
4 Inactivity of modern adult life.
5 Exposure to risk on the roads and at work.
6 Unemployment, divorce and other stressful life events.

Means of prevention

In this section we will discuss solely the specific preventive measures that should be taken to reduce the risk of disease in people aged between 25 and 64 years. The measures can be considered under two headings—health education and personal preventive services.

Chapter 7

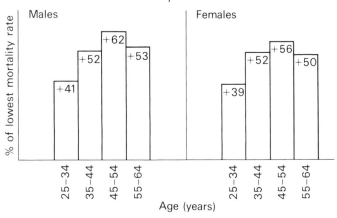

Fig. 7.2. Health improvement opportunities. Mortality in the U.K. expressed as a percentage of the lowest composite mortality rate of the U.S.A., Sweden, Canada and the U.K.

Health education

People in this group need to be given the opportunity to think about the risks they run and the means by which these risks can be reduced. This does not mean that they need be made neurotic about their health and life-style but they should be given the opportunity to think and discuss their options. Unfortunately, they are a difficult group to contact since, unlike young people, the majority do not regularly attend an educational setting, and there is little opportunity for reaching them. Many do attend adult education classes on health, e.g. they join the 'Look After Yourself' groups sponsored by the Health Education Council, but those who do are a self-selected group. In addition, some occupational health departments give advice on prevention, but for the majority education has to take place through two media.

1 One-to-one health education when a person consults his GP or health visitor (see p. 41).

2 Education through newspapers, radio and television.

It is, however, difficult to give a great deal of information or have protracted discussion using either of these media, and the most important means of health education of adults in the long term is the health education of children, so that they become better informed adults. Many of today's adults know very little about health, but tomorrow's adults should be much better informed. At present, one-to-one health education is the most influential, but it is difficult to discuss health issues with someone who has only a vague impression where his heart is, or what it does, or what is meant by the term dietary fat. Obviously the doctor or nurse has to adapt his delivery to suit the person he is addressing, but many people today are so ignorant of how their body works that an intelligent discussion about their health is difficult in the amount of time available for a consultation.

Personal preventive services
The 'annual check-up' (multiphasic screening) was at one time considered to be the best means of preventing disease in this age group. However, this has now been shown to be an inefficient means of preventing disease and the emphasis has swung to the development of specific detection and treatment programmes, each tailored to achieve one specific objective. The services that should be available for well people in this age group are few in number.
1 Family planning services.
2 Cervical cytology.
3 Regular measurement of blood pressure.
4 Regular tetanus boosters.
5 Regular dental inspection.
In addition, the person of this age group needs to be offered the opportunity to talk about his health; this can be done when he has made contact with his GP for advice about a symptom that is troubling him.

Women's problems

Although women have lower mortality rates than men at all ages there is growing interest in the provision of preventive services aimed specifically at women for the following reasons.
1 Disability and handicap are more common among women.
2 Certain women's health problems are more effectively tackled by a preventive approach, e.g. women are prescribed psychotropic drugs twice as often as men, not because they develop psychoses more often but because of the social factors which

influence self-referral and the social factors which influence medical management of problems which have social origins.

3 Certain women's diseases are preventable, notably cervical cancer.

4 Usually women are more interested in contraception than men are and thus contraceptive services are orientated towards women.

5 The lives of women are more affected by children than are the lives of men, particularly because of the growing numbers of divorces in which the woman is left as the head of a single parent family.

6 Women are, in general, poorer than men.

7 The life-style of women is changing and this has an effect on their health, e.g. the prevalence of smoking is increasing among women.

8 The growing number of women doctors in general practice.

For these reasons there is growing interest in the development of educational and preventive programmes for women, e.g.:

(i) 'Well women' clinics, organized by health visitors and GPs.

(ii) Community-based women's groups, both groups that focus on single problems, such as 'Weight Watchers' or Aerobics groups, or groups that are concerned with the whole range of women's problems.

(iii) Services offered by employers, e.g. Marks and Spencer, who employ large numbers of women.

CHAPTER 8
THE PROBLEMS OF OLD AGE

The objectives of prevention in old age are more concerned with the quality of life than with its prolongation. The principal objectives are:

1 to prevent unnecessary loss of functional ability;
2 to prevent a deterioration in the quality of life due to social problems or distressing symptoms such as pain or depression;
3 to prevent the breakdown of relatives;
4 to keep people in their own homes as long as possible.

Some of the problems that occur in old age cannot be prevented because they are caused by the ageing process; however, others can be prevented because they are the result of three other processes that cause problems in the elderly, i.e. disease, loss of fitness and social pressures. There is thus considerable scope for preventing the problems of old age. The 80-year-old person who has kept reasonably fit, who has been fortunate enough not to contract a disabling disease, and who has a good pension is able to cycle, garden, travel abroad, and enjoy life. The ageing process by itself does not cause significant disability until a very advanced age.

Prevention before old age

Prevention of the problems of the elderly has to start *before* old age if it is to be fully effective. Certain preventable childhood diseases have sequelae which affect health in old age (Table 8.1) and therefore the prevention of childhood problems will, many decades later, influence the health of the elderly population.

Similarly, an individual's health and life-style in adult life influence his health in old age. For example, the prevalence of cigarette smoking, obesity and inactivity in a population aged between 30 and 50 years of age will influence the numbers and health of that cohort when they are aged between 70 and 90.

Table 8.1. Diseases of childhood with long-term sequelae

Disease	Long-term sequelae
Poliomyelitis	Paralysis of major muscle groups
Tuberculosis	Impairment of lung and joint function
Rickets	Pelvis deformity resulting in obstetric difficulties resulting in stress incontinence
Rheumatic fever	Heart failure
Measles associated with malnutrition in an era in in which there were no antibiotics	The suppurative complications that can develop in those circumstances causes impairment of joint and lung function

Prevention in old age

However, there is still scope for prevention *in* old age because the problems of old people are not all due to the ageing process. A proportion are caused by those processes mentioned above—diseases, loss of fitness and social pressures.

Prevention of disease in old age

Certain diseases can be prevented by action taken after the age of 65 years. It is worth emphasizing that the commonest preventable disease in old age is iatrogenic disease caused in part by inappropriate medication, in part by inadequate communication and surveillance. It is sometimes suggested that the reason why old people make mistakes with their medication is the high prevalence of dementia in old age, but the principal responsibility for the prevention of such problems rests not with old people but with the medical profession.

Prevention of unfitness

For most people there is a steady loss of physical ability from about the age of 20 years onwards. In part this is due to the ageing process which leads to a loss in the maximum level of ability , but it is also due to the loss of fitness. In most people the gap between the actual level of ability and the best possible level of ability that he could attain were he fully fit—the fitness gap—widens with age (Fig. 8.1).

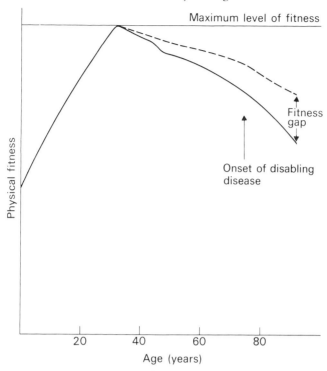

Fig. 8.1. Rate of change of physical fitness with age: rate of decline due to ageing alone if fitness is not lost (- - - -); actual rate of decline (——). (After Gray, J. A. M. (1982) *Brit. med. J.* **285**, 545–547.)

The rate at which a person loses fitness increases with age and the rate at which fitness is regained slows down, but the main reason why people lose fitness as they get older is social. There is a steady loss in the average amount of daily physical activity as we grow older because of the life-style that most people adopt in adult life. All four of the main aspects of fitness—strength, stamina, suppleness, and skill—are lost, but all can be regained by elderly people. The rate at which they can be regained is certainly slower the older the individual, but there is no upper age limit and, in general, older people can achieve a greater proportionate improvement in their level of ability by training than can young people, because the fitness gap is greater in old age due to the cumulative effect of inactivity.

The other important cause of loss of fitness is disabling disease; one effect of such diseases is to reduce the amount of physical activity a person takes, so that he enters a vicious cycle. Active leisure pursuits are obviously important in the prevention of this loss of fitness, but of great importance—especially for housebound elderly people—are the simple tasks of looking after themselves and their dwellings. Too often friends and relatives try to 'help' elderly people by taking over the very tasks which could keep them fit. Old people have a right to be at risk and a right to struggle, and the old person who continues to look after him/herself, even though it is a bit of a struggle and they are at risk in doing so, is keeping fit and healthy.

Prevention of social problems
Certain social problems are more common among elderly people, notably housing difficulties, poverty and isolation. Elderly people who are immobile, have dementia, or who have communication problems obviously have difficulty in claiming social security and in maintaining their house. But the basic cause of the social problem of older people is low income, and this reflects the attitudes of society towards old age and the political weakness of elderly people who are, as yet, insufficiently organized to exert political influence.

Primary prevention

Primary prevention in old age is the most effective form of approach but, as at any age, it is the most difficult and expensive to achieve. The education of elderly people, starting before retirement and continuing throughout life, together with their helpers is obviously important but education by itself will not be effective in preventing the problems faced by elderly people. The provision of adequate pensions, of well designed housing and of a good system of public transport are equally important measures which are, however, much more expensive than an educational programme; so it is not surprising that it is the latter which forms the central component in any programme of primary prevention.

Secondary prevention

Much of the debate about screening in old age has been confused because of the failure to distinguish between screening—the detection of asymptomatic disease—and case-finding, which is the detection of problems which were bothering the old person but were previously unreported. Many tests have been suggested as being effective in the detection of asymptomatic disease in old age. These range from the measurement of blood pressure to the measurement of intraocular pressure, but some of these tests have proved to be ineffective in achieving any of the objectives listed at the beginning of this chapter. Case-finding, on the other hand, does improve the quality of life of many elderly people (i) because it allows some of the problems that the old person had previously not even reported to the health or social services to be detected and solved, (ii) because many elderly people find it reassuring and encouraging to have someone take an interest in them.

For these reasons it can be argued that every person over the age of 75 should be contacted annually by someone from the health or social services. This would not be a very expensive task since the majority of old people initiate a contact at least once a year, leaving only a minority who should be identified and visited to see if any new problems have developed since the last contact.

Tertiary prevention

The ageing process reduces the body's ability to respond to challenges quickly and appropriately, and reduces the powers of repair and recovery. Elderly people are therefore more adversely affected by disease, and the active and effective management of acute and chronic disease is of vital importance in (i) the prevention of physical deterioration and (ii) the achievement of the four objectives of health care in old age.

COMMON RISK FACTORS

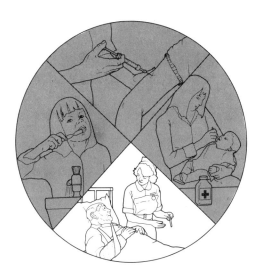

CHAPTER 9
EXERCISE IN PREVENTION

There are few data on the activity levels of people 40–80 years ago, but there is no doubt that people now are generally less active than they were in those times. The reasons are obvious: car ownership has increased and the energy expenditure required in the workplace and the home has decreased. There is, however, evidence that this decline has stopped and that there is now an increase in activity levels due to the increase in active leisure pursuits, notably cycling, running, jogging, aerobics and squash. This trend is welcome for there is increasing evidence that exercise can prevent disease and promote health.

Exercise in primary prevention

Regular physical exercise plays a part in the prevention of three common disorders—coronary heart disease, osteoporosis and obesity.

Coronary heart disease

The mechanisms by which exercise prevents coronary heart disease are unknown but four hypotheses are popular.

'1 An increase in physical activity leads to lower concentrations of triglycerides, very low density lipoprotein cholesterol, and low density lipoprotein cholesterol while, perhaps most importantly, increasing concentrations of high density lipoprotein cholesterol. Such alterations in blood lipid profiles are strongly related to a lower risk of coronary heart disease.

2 Physical conditioning augments a rise in fibrinolysis induced by venous occlusion and alters platelet stickiness and thrombus formation. Exercise may be implicated favourably in counteracting the pathophysiology of atherosclerotic processes.

3 Exercise adequate to achieve physical fitness has many salutary

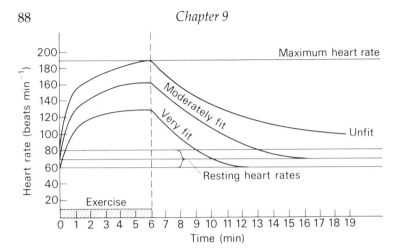

Fig. 9.1. The relationship between exercise, heart rate and fitness.

effects; it increases maximal oxygen uptake, slows the heart rate (Fig. 9.1), lowers blood pressure, decreases ventricular ectopic activity, increases maximal cardiac output, and increases physical work capacity.

4 Exercise increases insulin sensitivity and may be effective against insulin resistant states, such as obesity and maturity onset diabetes, both of which are implicated as risk factors in coronary heart disease.'

(Thomas, G. S., Lee, P. R., Franks, P. & Paffenberger, R. S. (1981) *Exercise and Health*, pp. 40, 41. Oelgeschlager, Gunn and Hain.)

Among people who have a high level of physical exercise at work the risk of heart disease is inversely related to the energy output (Fig. 9.2). Among those who have sedentary jobs the risk is inversely related to the amount of energy expended in leisure activities. A study of Harvard graduates showed that participation in vigorous sports offered protection against heart disease (Fig. 9.3). Another study of a sedentary population, that of British civil servants, also demonstrated that vigorous exercise was necessary for the prevention of coronary heart disease. The message is clear. To reduce the risk of heart disease it is essential to exercise sufficiently vigorously to become breathless and increase the heart rate sufficiently.

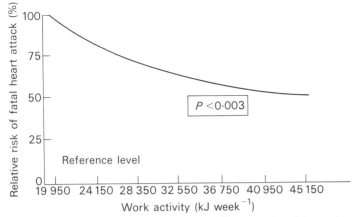

Fig. 9.2. Regression analysis of the relative risk of heart attack with increasing work activity. Risk of a fatal heart attack is progressively lowered to 50% as work energy output is doubled. (From Thomas, G. S. *et al.* (1981) *Exercise and Health.* Oelgeschlager, Gunn and Hain.)

In addition to the primary prevention of coronary heart disease, physical exercise can also reduce the risk of recurrence among those who have had one heart attack.

Obesity

Control of energy intake is central to any programme of weight

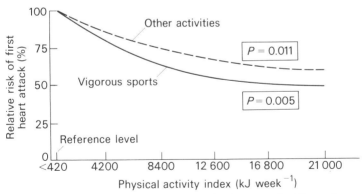

Fig. 9.3. Regression analysis of relative risk of first heart attack in Harvard students over a 6–10 year follow-up. Reduced risk of heart attack is seen with increasing energy output from each type of activity, but at any given level of output the risk is far lower for vigorous sports play. (From Thomas, G. S. *et al.* (1981) *Exercise and Health.* Oelgeschlager, Gunn and Hain.)

control, but increased energy expenditure by physical exercise also has a very important part to play in weight control. The formula is simple.

1 kg of body fat = 31.570 kJ
Walking 1 mile = 328 kJ
∴ Walking 96 miles = 1 kg of body fat
In half an hour one can walk 2 miles
In a year one can walk 730 miles by walking half an hour a day
∴ Walking half an hour a day for a year will be equal to 7.6 kg
   leading to a loss of 7.6 kg (16.7 lb) of fat.

Osteoporosis

The effects of complete immobilization on bone are well recognized: there is demineralization and loss of bone. The effects of partial immobilization are also now recognized, in part due to the interest in weightlessness stimulated by the space programme. The fact that most old people do not use their limbs fully and do not bear weight as much as they did when younger contributes to the osteoporosis (i.e. bone atrophy) and therefore contributes to one of our modern epidemics—fractured neck of femur.

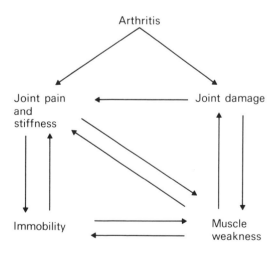

Fig. 9.4. The vicious circle of immobility.

Exercise in tertiary prevention

It is now appreciated that the loss of function that takes place in many diseases is due not only to the primary effects of the disease on the affected tissues but also to the effects of immobility. Physical exercise is beneficial in the following diseases:
1 maturity-onset diabetes mellitus;
2 peripheral vascular disease;
3 mildly high blood pressure;
4 chronic obstructive airways disease;
5 diseases that impair joint mobility, e.g. arthritis, stroke and Parkinson's disease;
6 asthma.
Exercise is particularly beneficial in old age (see p. 81).

Hazards of exercise

A patient with a disease is usually prepared to accept the risks of treatment because he has no other option, but the encouragement of healthy people to take up an activity that carries a risk, no matter how small, poses difficult problems. The hazards involved therefore have to be taken into account when promoting exercise.

Coronary hazards
The risk is small but it does exist and people need advice on the means by which such risks can be minimized.

Isometric exercise carries a higher risk than isotonic because of its effects on blood pressure and myocardial oxygen consumption. A combination of isometric and isotonic exercise is particularly dangerous, for example carrying a heavy suitcase and walking quickly. The person who is unfit or who has several coronary risk factors should therefore be advised to avoid this type of exercise and to avoid highly competitive sports such as squash.

Medical assessment is not necessary for everyone who wishes to take more exercise but people who have any of the following characteristics should be advised to consult their GP.
1 obesity;
2 cigarette smoking;

3 the presence of heart disease, high blood pressure, chest pains, or cardiac arrhythmias;

4 having a close relative who had a stroke or heart attack under the age of 50.

In addition, anyone who has a chronic disease requiring treatment should consult their doctor. But there is no evidence that the 'exercise ECG', namely an ECG taken when the individual is taking exercise, is effective in identifying high risk individuals.

Everyone who takes up active leisure pursuits should be advised to build up gently and gradually and seek help if they suffer pain or severe distress.

Musculo-skeletal overuse syndromes

These are legion and the precise syndrome depends on the parts of the body used, e.g. joggers and runners suffer problems in the lower limbs. However, many of these problems are preventable by:

1 proper training, with particular emphasis on suppleness;

2 proper warming up;

3 proper kit and equipment;

4 proper advice at an early stage by an interested doctor or physiotherapist should injury occur.

Accidents and sporting injuries

These are real risks but many injuries and accidents can be prevented by sensible training and warming up, the use of appropriate kit or equipment, and strict refereeing in body-contact sports.

Action

Education

It is important to correct mistaken beliefs and to provide information about the health benefits of exercise. It seems probable, however, that the desire to participate in exercise is at least as likely to be in response to fashion as it is to indicate a desire to prevent disease. As a first step it is necessary to improve the education of professionals so that they prescribe safe, effective and enjoyable exercise. General exhortations are less helpful than specific advice. The average person requires specific guidance on four aspects of the exercise.

1 Type of exercise.
2 Duration.
3 Intensity.
4 Frequency.

Social action

There is also a need for action by local and central government, such as those provisions listed in Table 9.1 with the authority responsible and the source of finance.

Sports Councils have an important part to play nationally and, at local level, a number of different local authority departments are involved. However, the rate of development of these

Table 9.1. Actions to facilitate exercise.

Action	Responsibility	Source of finance
More cycle tracks	Highways authorities, e.g. County Councils	Rates
More sport and leisure centres	Central government Private developers also interested, especially in squash	Sports Council grants Central government grants ('Urban Aid')
Provision of a shower in every place of work	None at present; could be added to legal requirements using the Health and Safety at Work Act 1974	Employers can at present claim tax relief on sports facilities for employees
Open school facilities to community	Local education authority	Rates—the cost is small, covered in part by charges
Employment of community-based physical education teachers	Local education authority Local authority recreation departments	Rates
Development of classes in aerobics, jazz dancing, keep fit, etc.	Local education authority Local authority recreation departments	Rates—cost covered in part by charges Private enterprise now active in aerobics

Chapter 9

facilities could be increased if the medical profession were to emphasize more strongly that physical exercise is not simply a pastime but an important means of disease prevention.

CHAPTER 10
POVERTY AND EQUALITY

Two types of poverty are recognized by economists:

absolute poverty when a person has insufficient wealth to buy the necessities of life, e.g. food, water or shelter;

relative poverty when he has insufficient wealth to buy what most people in his society regard as being necessary for an enjoyable life-style, not a luxurious one but one that is relatively free from financial strain, e.g. in the U.K. a car, new clothes from time to time, a holiday once a year, a visit to the cinema or theatre and good housing.

In developed countries social security systems exist which are intended to prevent absolute poverty, although many people on the lowest level of social security are unable to afford adequate housing and may thus be considered to be in absolute poverty. The absolute levels of income of these people who are in receipt of social security is therefore of relevance in disease prevention and health promotion. The effects of low income, and all its consequences, can be most clearly investigated by considering the health of poor people, relative to the health of those who are better off, i.e. by considering the effects of relative poverty. However, it is customary not simply to consider differences in health in different income groups but to group people by social class, that is in groups with similar amounts of resources and life-styles, taking occupation as the indicator of social class. Imperfect though this approach may be, it is the method used by the Registrar General, who recognizes five classes, now usually known as occupational classes rather than social classes:

I   Professional, e.g. doctor, lawyer (5%).

II   Intermediate, e.g. nurse, schoolteacher (18%)

IIIN Skilled non-manual, e.g. secretary, shop assistant (12%).

IIIM Skilled manual, e.g. bus driver, carpenter, coal-face worker (38%).

IV   Partly skilled, e.g. agricultural worker, postman (18%).

V   Unskilled, e.g. cleaner, dock worker, labourer (9%).

Impact of poverty and inequality

There are a number of trends that can easily be observed when health statistics are grouped according to occupational class:

1 Mortality rates increase from class I to IV (Fig. 10.1). This increase is particularly marked in childhood (see p. 55) but persists throughout life.

2 The incidence of low birth weight babies increases from class I to V.

3 The prevalence of chronic disease and disability increases from class I to V (Table 10.1).

4 Although there is an increase in the rate of health service utilization from class I to V there are services which are relatively under used, particularly preventive services.

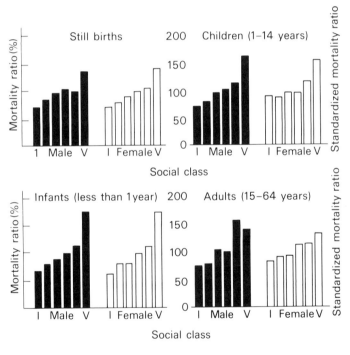

Fig. 10.1. Mortality by occupational class and age. Relative mortality (%) is the ratio of rates for one occupational class to the rate for all males or females (After Townsend, P. & Davidson, N. (1982) *Inequalities in Health* (The Black Report). Penguin Books, Harmondsworth, Middlesex.)

Table 10.1. Sickness and medical consultation in early adulthood (average rates per 1 000 population 1971–6)* (After Townsend, P. & Davidson, N. (1982) *Inequalities in Health* (The Black Report). Penguin Books, Harmondsworth, Middlesex.)

Socio-economic group	Limited long-standing illness		Restricted activity (in two-week period)		Consultations	
	Males	Females	Males	Females	Males	Females[†]
Professional	79	81	78	89	105	134
Managerial	119	115	74	83	113	137
Intermediate	143	140	83	95	116	155
Skilled manual	141	135	87	86	123	147
Semi-skilled manual	168	203	87	102	131	160
Unskilled manual	236	257	101	103	153	158
Ratio unskilled manual to professional	3.0	3.2	1.3	1.2	1.5	1.2

* England and Wales for 1971–2.
[†] 1972–6.

The most worrying trend is the secular trend—for there is no evidence that the gap between the classes is decreasing. Indeed, there is evidence that the gap is actually increasing.

Relative importance of poverty
There is now good evidence that the differences in the prevalence of poverty can explain most of the differences in health observed between people in different racial groups or geographical regions.

Feasibility of prevention

It has been argued that the differences in health of people in different occupational groups reflect genetic or biological differences between the groups but there is no evidence that this is so. Poverty appears to be the main factor. It has been demonstrated in Sweden that the difference in health associated with poverty can be eliminated. Striking evidence is provided by a comparative study of five counties in Sweden, three of which were formerly poorer than the others (Fig. 10.2). The trend in the last

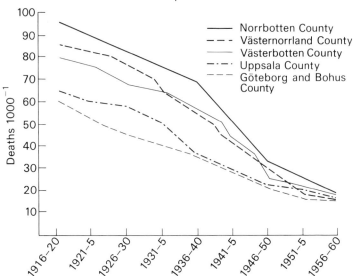

Fig. 10.2. Infant mortality in five Swedish counties, 1916–60. (After Townsend, P. & Davidson, N. (1982) *Inequalities of Health* (The Black Report). Penguin Books, Harmondsworth, Middlesex.)

40 years has been for the difference in infant mortality between the rich counties and the poor counties to disappear.

It is, however, important to try to identify the specific factors that are responsible for the higher incidence of disease among poor people. This may allow the development of policies that will modify these factors and bring about a more rapid reduction in the incidence of disease than will be brought about by general policies aimed at the elimination of poverty. Three factors are of particular importance: the physical environment, working conditions, and life-style.

Physical environment
Poor people live in worse housing conditions and the environment in which their housing is set is also more likely to be harmful to health.

Working conditions
Obviously the jobs done by poor people expose them to a greater risk of accident and disease.

Life-style

This is the most important factor. From class I to class V the following important differences in life-style occur.

1 Increasing prevalence of cigarette smoking.

2 Decreasing participation in active leisure pursuits.

3 Increasing consumption of fats, refined carbohydrate and decreasing consumption of fruit and wholemeal bread.

In part this is due to the differences in income levels of people in different classes, but there are other more important factors that have to be taken into account:

1 Poor people living in conditions of uncertainty are less likely to be influenced by educational messages about benefits 20 or 30 years in the future.

2 People who are rejected by employers and given only a survival wage by society may come to regard themselves with less esteem and therefore care less about their bodies than those people who are highly rewarded by society.

3 Those who are made redundant or homeless, or whose lives are determined largely by forces over which they have no control, are less likely to believe that they can influence the probability that they will die or become disabled than wealthy people who have a much larger degree of control of their housing conditions, their working life and place of residence.

It is not sufficient simply to offer poor people more information. Their health problems and their beliefs and attitudes have to be considered in the context of their economic and social position.

Risk reduction

There are two approaches to the prevention of diseases caused by poverty:

1 Specific measures designed to tackle the consequences of poverty.

2 General measures to prevent poverty.

Specific measures

Being poor has certain consequences that increase the risk of disease and these can be tackled, although the measures used at present are relatively ineffective (Table 10.2).

Table 10.2.

Consequences of poverty	Specific measures used at present	Limitations	Ideal measures
Insufficient income	Maintenance of social-security payments in line with inflation Provision of extra financial benefits for groups most in need, i.e. children, pregnant women and disabled people	Increases in social security always lag behind increases in the cost of living Low uptake of special benefits by those eligible for them	Increase in real value of social security Simplification of social security system Real increase in value of old-age pension
Unhealthy physical environment	Building of new local-authority dwellings Renovation of old dwellings Urban redevelopment Reduction of lead in petrol	Provision of cheap housing may merely create a different set of problems, e.g. problems of high-rise blocks Housing is a low priority in the U.K. Some groups, e.g. single people under pension age, are not recognized by local authorities	Removal of lead from petrol Increased investment in housing

Dangerous working conditions	Implementation of Health and Safety at Work Act	Unwillingness of employers to act	New attitude towards occupational health by employers and by the medical profession
Inadequate utilization of health services	Development of primary health care. Increased attention given to the organization of services to meet the needs of people without cars. Investment of extra resources in areas in which poverty is more prevalent	Lack of resources for health-service development. Gap between health authority and family practitioner committee planning. Lack of consumer participation. Gaps between health authority and local authority planning	A real commitment to the development of primary health care
Unhealthy life-style	Increased interest in health education	Present style still based too strongly on assumption that people are ignorant and simply need to be told what to do	Development of a participative style of education which is concerned not only with health risks but with the economic and political determinants of health

General measures

These specific measures, important though they are, should not divert attention from the fact that the main aim must be to reduce the prevalence of poverty. There are two opposing approaches to the prevention of poverty—the creation or redistribution of national wealth. Those who believe in the former believe that society should devote its energies to the creation of wealth so that all social classes will become wealthier; the latter believe that steps should be taken to redistribute the wealth that we have. The difference of opinion is aggravated by the fact that the former group also believe that the steps a government must take to redistribute wealth—i.e. increased taxation, additional borrowing and growth in public expenditure—create inflation and prevent the creation of wealth.

These are economic and political questions but it could be argued that it is as important to tackle inequality as it is to tackle poverty, because the culture that develops among a group of people who feel rejected and unimportant is one in which poor health is accepted as normal and inevitable.

CHAPTER 11
NUTRITION

Introduction

It is ironic that, in Western societies, while dietary changes probably contributed as much as any other factor to improvements in
health in the first half of the twentieth century, faulty diets
should be a cause of so much ill-health in the second half of the
century. The improvements were generally due to correction of
'deficiencies', in both the quality and quantity of food eaten by
most of the population. Conversely, the harmful effects now are
the consequences of 'excesses', again both qualitative and quanti-
tative. However, while this is of course true of urbanized, industrialized societies, it should not be forgotten that for a large part of
the world dietary deficiencies remain the nutritional problem.

Historical background

Scurvy
The history of nutritional disorders is largely concerned with the
association of dietary deficiencies with illness. The well known
observation (probably the first 'controlled trial'!) by James Lind in
1753 that scurvy, a major disability amongst sailors on long
voyages, could be cured—and prevented—by the juice of citrus
fruits, established the concept of deficiency diseases for the first
time. Interestingly, it was not until more than a century and a half
later that the active agent, vitamin C, was isolated and identified.

Early twentieth century
In 1904 an influential report of the Inter-Departmental Committee on Physical Deterioration (set up because of the poor
physical state of those volunteering for the Boer War) disclosed
serious under-nutrition in the population, due to poverty. This
initiated a number of major social reforms, including not only the
establishment of National Health Insurance, Old Age Pensions

and Unemployment Benefit, but also the provision of school milk and school meals, at least to a limited extent.

In a further early 'controlled trial' in a London orphanage in the 1920s, supplementation of the diet with a daily pint of milk was shown to result in taller, heavier, more lively children. Milk came to be seen as an important high-quality food which provided a significant addition, particularly of protein and calcium, to an inadequate diet. About the same time, bone deformities due to rickets—a common disorder in children, especially in urban populations—was shown to be prevented and cured by vitamin D, and cod-liver oil began to enjoy a vogue.

Many surveys in the 1920s and 1930s showed that children attending fee-paying schools were better nourished, taller and heavier than their contemporaries attending State schools. It was also known that the average height and weight of people living in the country was greater than that of those living in towns. There was also a correlation between social class and height, low socio-economic status being associated with low stature which, although partly genetic, was also an indicator of past nutrition. This is much less evident than it was but the relatively impaired growth of some women of lower social class is a contributory factor to the higher perinatal mortality in this sector of the population.

Nevertheless, there was a continual increase in the stature of men and women at the turn of the century (Fig. 11.1) and this (together with improvements in sanitation and housing) was associated with a decline in disease, especially tuberculosis.

Second World War

Surprisingly perhaps, the outbreak in 1939 of the Second World War with the consequent threat to food supplies, 'rationing' and special allowances for mothers and children, led to adequate provision of essential foods for more of the population than previously and hence improvements in general nutrition. Welfare foods included milk, cod-liver oil and orange juice, margarine was fortified with vitamins A and D, and a higher extraction brown flour (containing more iron, vitamin B and fibre) was used for bread. Perinatal mortality during the War

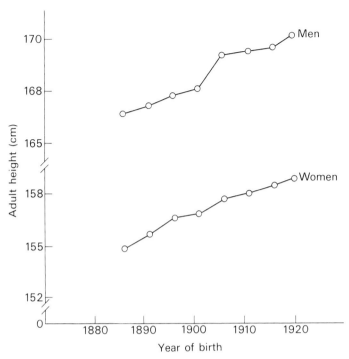

Fig. 11.1. Attained height of British adults born at different times. All figures are the mean for 5-year age groups, except those for 1920 which are based on a 3-year group. (After DHSS (1979) *Prevention and Health: Eating for Health*. HMSO, London.)

years showed one of its steepest falls ever, and the height of those born during the 1940s was substantially greater than that of people born in the previous decade.

The present time
Subsequently, increasing affluence and the availability of an even greater variety of foods has meant that, in our society, concern is now with the ill-effects of 'over-nutrition', rather than of undernourishment or dietary deficiency. In contrast with the relatively simple and dramatic correction of deficiency disorders which occurred once their cause was known, the correction of disorders of over-nutrition seems to pose a much more complex and tedious problem.

Diseases of Affluence

These are the diseases characteristic of Western urbanized industrial societies which seem to be rare or absent in the Third World, though assuming more significance in those countries which are 'developing' on Western lines. They include ischaemic heart disease, diabetes, gall-stones, diverticular disease of the colon, irritable bowel syndrome, constipation, appendicitis, large bowel cancer, haemorrhoids, varicose veins, dental caries and last, but not least, obesity.

Western diet
This is thought to contribute substantially to these diseases and several aspects of the typical Western diet have been incriminated. Such a diet is characterized by a preponderance of fatty foods, of foods with a high sugar and low fibre content, and by an excess of alcohol. Moreover, three-quarters of food eaten in the U.K. is 'processed' at least once, which alters the composition and makes identification of ingredients difficult (a task which is not eased by poor labelling). The Western diet commonly includes high proportions of sweets, cakes, biscuits, butter, margarine, cream, cooking fats and fried foods. Less bread is eaten than formerly and most of this is made from white flour (though there is an encouraging recent increase in the proportion of wholemeal bread consumed). Total energy intake is generally excessive and so usually is the amount of salt eaten.

During this century the proportion of protein in the diet has remained roughly the same, though in the last two or three decades the proportion of this derived from meat has increased from about one-half to almost two-thirds.

The proportion of carbohydrate has fallen by about one-third because, although there has been an increase in dietary sugar, less bread and fewer potatoes are eaten (Figs 11.2 and 11.3).

But the dietary change which causes most concern is the increase in fat, which now contributes about 42% of total energy intake. Moreover, more than three-quarters of this, being derived from meat and dairy products, is of the 'saturated fatty acid' variety. However, there has been some recent change here: the ratio of polyunsaturated to saturated fatty acids have in-

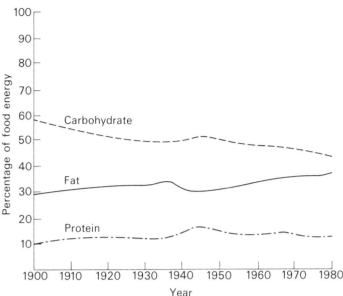

Fig. 11.2. Changes in the twentieth century in the proportion of dietary carbohydrates, fat and protein consumed as a percentage of food energy. (After DHSS (1979) *Prevention and Health: Eating for Health*. HMSO, London.)

creased slightly because of a decrease in the consumption of butter and an increase in that of margarine and cooking oils over the last few years.

One important component of Western diet which must not be forgotten is alcohol. The proportion of this has doubled in the last 20 years and it now represents about 5% of energy intake. Moreover, the problems associated with this increase are of course not limited to the nutritional field (see Chapter 13).

One characteristic of Western diets which has received increased attention recently is its deficiency in 'dietary fibre'. This rather misleading term refers to complex, non-absorbable carbohydrates. These are present in various foods but that of cereal origin seems to be particularly important. When its importance was first suggested by Cleeve, no interest was taken, but it is now thought that dietary fibre may be important not only in the prevention of bowel disorders but of other diseases too.

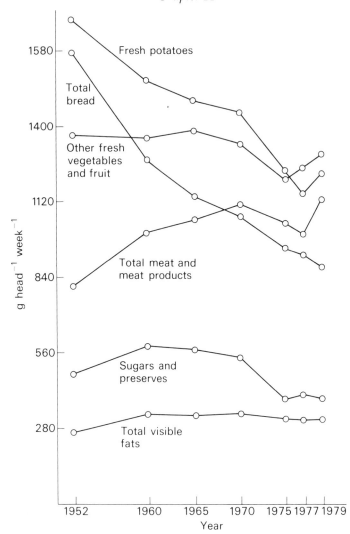

Fig. 11.3. Average household consumption of some groups of foods 1952–79. (After Ministry of Agriculture, fisheries and food. Annual Reports of the National Food Survey Committee, 1954 onwards. HMSO, London.)

Relationship between diet and disease

There is accumulating evidence, mostly from epidemiological sources, of the association between Western diet and disease. The evidence has been of various kinds. Different countries with substantially different dietary habits have markedly different incidences of diseases which seem difficult to account for in other ways; and populations moving from one country to another and acquiring the dietary habits of the new country also tend to acquire that country's diseases. Moreover, within a given country, individuals with dietary habits differing from the norm, e.g. vegetarians, also have different disease patterns. In relation to certain diseases changes with known risk factors are associated with changes in diet. Finally, in a few cases, controlled trials, particularly difficult as these are, have recently demonstrated a relationship between diet and disease.

Coronary heart disease
This is the major killer in industrial societies. In an early study of the relation between diet and deaths from ischaemic heart disease in seven countries, Keys* showed that there were strong positive correlations between the amount of saturated fat and dietary sugar eaten, blood cholesterol concentrations and deaths from coronary heart disease. Other studies showed that migrating populations, e.g. Japanese moving to California, in adopting a higher fat diet also acquired a higher incidence of ischaemic heart disease. More recently, the results of intervention studies such as the Oslo Heart Study, a controlled trial in which dietary and smoking advice were studied, have shown a reduction in coronary heart deaths in men who reduced their fat intake. There has been much debate about the relative importance of 'saturated' and 'polyunsaturated' fats. The evidence indicates that it is a high fat intake which is harmful and particularly a high intake of saturated fat.

There is also evidence that a high alcohol intake is associated with coronary heart disease but, although a high intake of sugar is harmful for many reasons, there is little support for the view that excess dietary sugar may contribute directly.

Hypertension
This is a common condition in industrial societies and a major risk for cardiovascular disease, particularly strokes and coronary

*Keys, A. (1980) *Seven Countries: A Multivariate Analysis of Death and Coronary Heart Disease*. Harvard University Press, Cambridge.

heart disease. There is an association with obesity, and losing weight leads to a fall in blood pressure. There is also a correlatio: between salt intake and high blood pressure, evidence that a high salt intake may cause hypertension, at least in susceptible individuals, and further evidence that reducing salt intake may reverse the process.

Diabetes
Diet plays an important part in the aetiology of 'maturity-onset' (non insulin – dependent) diabetes. Its incidence correlates strongly with an excessive energy intake. High-fibre diets have now been shown to improve the control of diabetes and a high-fibre diet may help to protect against the development of maturity-onset diabetes.

Diverticular disease
This condition is more or less exclusive to those eating a Western-type diet and is almost unknown in countries where diets are rich in cereal foods and contain little fat or sugar. Studies in this country have confirmed that a high fibre intake helps to protect against diverticular disease and that treatment with bran provides symptomatic relief for those suffering from it. Vegetarians are much less prone to diverticular disease than others and a dietary fibre intake of about 30 g a day seems important.

Constipation and irritable bowel syndrome
These are also common complaints in Western society and rare in countries with high fibre diets and in vegetarians. Increasing dietary fibre increases stool bulk, reduces bowel transit times and relieves constipation and irritable bowel symptoms.

Gall-stones and appendicitis
Both these conditions occur more frequently in those on diets deficient in fibre. Gall-stones are also associated with obesity.

Cancer
Various cancers are attributable to aspects of diet. In a recent report Doll and Peto* estimated that about one-third of all deaths from cancer are attributable to diet, about the same proportion as those caused by smoking. Epidemiological evidence indicates

*Doll, R. & Peto, R. (1981) *The Causes of Cancer.* Oxford University Press, Oxford.

that diet may be important in determining the occurrence of cancer of the stomach, large bowel, uterus (body), gall bladder and liver. It may also contribute to cancer of the breast and pancreas. The mechanisms are unclear, but there is some evidence that dietary fat may be implicated and that the vitamin A precursor beta-carotene may be protective.

Dental caries

This is a major problem in the U.K. and has been for a long time. Its incidence in children is strongly related to sugar consumption and restricted supplies of sugar during the Second World War led to improvements in the dental health of children, only for the situation to deteriorate again when sugar became freely available afterwards.

In a recent survey, 80% of 5-year-olds required treatment for dental caries, and in 10% more than half their teeth were seriously decayed. Caries is rare in countries where food is unrefined. The presence of one part per million of fluoride in drinking water also protects against dental decay.

Obesity

This is the commonest nutritional disorder in the U.K. and is an important cause of ill-health. It increases morbidity and mortality from a number of diseases and shortens life expectancy. Life Insurance data (Fig. 11.4) illustrate the risk to life.

Obesity arises when energy intake is in excess of expenditure and is usually the result of a long-term sustained slight excessive intake rather than temporary gourmandizing. Loss of excess weight requires not only the elimination of excess food consumption, but also a further reduction sufficient to compensate for the excess which caused the obesity. So in this instance prevention is clearly easier than cure.

Although exercise is important in the prevention of obesity, its importance relative to diet is often exaggerated (Table 11.1).

However, the relationship between energy intake and expenditure and obesity is a complex one. Energy needs seem to vary considerably. This is because of differences not only in physical activity, but also in basic metabolic requirements.

Chapter 11

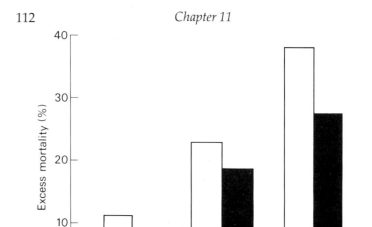

Fig. 11.4. Excess mortality among overweight men (□) and women (■) aged 15–69 years compared with all persons insured at standard risks. (After DHSS (1979). *Prevention and Health: Eating for Health.* HMSO, London.)

Table 11.1. Some food intakes and some physical activities which are equivalent in energy value to approximately 1260 kJ*.

Energy expenditure of 1260 kJ		Energy intake of 1260 kJ	
Activity	Time period	Food	Approximate quantity
Golf	2 h	Sugar	2¾ oz (75 g) or 18 lumps
Tennis	¾ to 1 h	Bread	6 slices
Gardening	¾ to 1 h	Milk	¾ pint (0.43 l)
Football	30–40 min	Cheese	2½ oz (70 g)
Competitive		Bacon	3 oz (84 g)
swimming/cross-		Eggs	3 large size
country running/	Less than	Potatoes	1 lb (0.45 kg)
hill-climbing	1 h	Biscuits	6 digestive biscuits
4-mile walk	1 h	Gin or Whisky	6 singles
Do-it-yourself		Beer	2 pints (1.14 l)
house repairs and	2 h	Table wine	0.50 l (2 glasses)
decorating			

* 1260 kJ is approximately the difference in energy expenditure between sedentary and moderately active occupations.

Dietary recommendations

These should be applicable to the population as a whole and should not be seen as aimed solely at vulnerable or 'at risk' individuals or groups. The purpose is the promotion of health and the primary prevention of disease, particularly those diseases listed above. Recommendations should be suitable for all age groups with minor modifications for certain categories of individuals and some specific recommendations for babies.

Dietary advice must be concerned with the broad composition of the total diet in terms of protein, fat, carbohydrate, etc., but should at the same time be specific in terms of foodstuffs. Wherever possible, advice should be reinforced and supplemented with simple literature. An example of appropriate literature is the 'natural diet' (Appendix 1). Free supplies of simple literature on diets may be obtained from Health Education Units or from the Health Education Council or Scottish Health Education Group (addresses at the end of this chapter).

The most important objective is to maintain weight within 10% of the 'ideal' or 'optimal' since this weight (obtained from Life Insurance data) is that associated with the lowest level of mortality. Table 11.2, derived from Metropolitan Life Insurance statistics, is a useful guide to the desired weight range. An alternative method of ascertaining an optimal or 'target' weight is to calculate the body mass index (BMI). This is the ratio of weight (kg) over the square of height (m). It should be 20–25 for men and 19–24 for women.

As discussed above, energy requirements vary greatly with individuals and are not only related to activity. Regular weighing is a necessary discipline for most people if obesity is to be controlled and many find participation in a 'slimming group' which incorporates regular weighing as well as other relevant activities helpful.

Advice on individual dietary constituents should include the following:

Sugar. The average individual's annual intake of sucrose is about 45 kg. About half of it is added to beverages, cereals, etc. The amount should be halved.

Fat. Many international and national, professional and

Table 11.2. Optimal weight for height. (After Consumers' Association (1978) *Which? Way to Slim.* Consumers' Association, London.)

Metric

	Height without shoes (cm)	Mean −10% (kg)	Mean for medium build (kg)	Mean +10% (kg)	Mean +20% (kg)
Men	155	49	54	59	64
	157	50	55	61	66
	160	51	57	63	68
	162	52	58	64	69
	165	54	60	66	71
	167	55	62	68	74
	170	57	64	70	76
	172	59	65	72	78
	175	60	67	74	80
	177	63	69	76	83
	180	64	71	79	85
	183	66	74	80	88

Imperial

	Height without shoes ft ins	Mean −10% st lb	Mean for medium build st lb	Mean +10% st lb	Mean +20% st lb
Men	5 1	7 9	8 7	9 4	10 2
	5 2	7 12	8 10	9 8	10 6
	5 3	8 1	8 13	9 11	10 10
	5 4	8 3	9 2	10 1	10 13
	5 5	8 7	9 6	10 4	11 3
	5 6	8 10	9 10	10 9	11 8
	5 7	9 0	10 0	11 0	12 0
	5 8	9 4	10 4	11 4	12 4
	5 9	9 7	10 8	11 9	12 9
	5 10	9 11	10 13	12 0	13 1
	5 11	10 2	11 3	12 5	13 6
	6 0	10 6	11 8	12 9	13 11

Metric (height in cm; weights in kg)

Height				
186	68	75	83	90
188	70	78	85	93
191	72	80	88	96

Women

Height				
142	40	45	49	54
145	41	46	51	55
147	43	47	52	56
150	44	49	54	58
152	45	50	55	60
155	46	51	56	61
157	48	53	58	63
160	49	55	60	65
162	51	57	63	68
165	52	59	64	70
167	54	61	66	72
170	57	63	68	74
172	58	64	70	76
175	59	66	72	79
177	61	68	74	81

Imperial (height in ft in; weights in st lb)

Height				
6 1	10 10	11 12	13 0	14 3
6 2	10 14	12 3	13 6	14 9
6 3	11 5	12 8	13 11	15 0

Women

Height				
4 8	6 5	7 1	7 10	8 6
4 9	6 7	7 3	7 13	8 9
4 10	6 10	7 6	8 2	8 12
4 11	6 12	7 9	8 6	9 2
5 0	7 1	7 12	8 9	9 6
5 1	7 4	8 1	8 12	9 9
5 2	7 7	8 5	9 2	9 13
5 3	7 10	8 8	9 6	10 4
5 4	8 0	8 13	9 11	10 9
5 5	8 4	9 3	10 1	11 0
5 6	8 7	9 7	10 6	11 5
5 7	8 11	9 11	10 10	11 9
5 8	9 1	10 1	11 0	12 0
5 9	9 4	10 5	11 5	12 5
5 10	9 8	10 9	11 9	12 10

All weights with indoor clothes, no shoes.

governmental committees have shown a strong consensus in the belief that lowering total fat in the diet to about 30% of total energy intake (from the current 40% or more) can reduce the risk of coronary heart disease. There is now also general agreement that effort should be concentrated on reducing saturated-fat intake in particular.

Fibre. Dietary fibre, particularly cereal fibre, is of special value. To its virtue as a laxative can now be added other probable benefits. An intake of about 30 g a day from foodstuffs derived from wholegrain cereals is recommended. Increased consumption of fruit and vegetables should also be encouraged.

Protein. The intake of protein in the U.K. has remained remarkably stable this century, despite other major dietary changes. Although average dietary protein intake exceeds requirement, there is no evidence suggesting changes are necessary; though eating less meat as a source of protein and more cereals and vegetables would, incidentally, reduce intake of saturated fat.

Salt. The present average salt intake of 12 g a day is excessive and could be halved without detriment and with possible benefits in preventing hypertension.

Alcohol. During the past 20 years alcohol consumption in the U.K. has doubled. To preserve health, alcohol intake should not exceed 4% of total calories, which means about 20 g or 2 'units' a day—the equivalent of two pints of beer or two glasses of wine or measures of spirits.

Dietary guidelines
In 1978 the Department of Health and Social Security in the U.K. published recommendations for the whole population. These may be summarized as follows.

1 A variety of foods should be eaten.

2 Obesity should be avoided.

3 Many people would benefit from modifying the balance of their overall diet by: (a) eating less fatty and sugary foods; (b) eating less salt; (c) drinking less alcohol; (d) eating more bread, potatoes and other vegetables and fruit.

4 Babies should be breast-fed if possible, even if only for a short time.

5 Growing children, teenagers, expectant and nursing mothers, and those who are house-bound may need additional vitamin D6. To make sure of a supply of all the essential nutrients the diet should comprise a mixture of foods from five food groups: (a) cereals; (b) milk and dairy foods; (c) fruit and vegetables; (d) fat and oils; (e) meat, fish, etc; and (f) non-dairy fat and oils.

Implementation

Providing advice and guide-lines is one thing. Putting them into effect is another. There are many obstacles to the effective implementation of dietary guide-lines because eating habits are influenced by a large number of factors, not least likes and dislikes. More research is required into the effectiveness of different ways of improving compliance with sensible dietary advice, but it is likely that personalized advice from an individual's GP is at least as effective as any other method.

Appendix 1

Eat plenty of fibre-containing foods
Wholemeal bread, wholemeal biscuits, crispbreads, oat cakes, Weetabix, Puffed Wheat, All Bran, whole wheat flakes, porridge, brown rice, wholemeal pasta
Fruit—always eat the skin
Vegetables, especially corn-on-the-cob, peas, lentils, baked beans, dried beans, e.g. butter beans, haricot and mexican beans
Jacket potatoes—always eat the skin
Always cook with wholemeal flour
Extend smaller quantities of meat, fish and cheese by using recipes which combine these with cereals and vegetables, e.g. casseroles

Eat less fatty food
Use skimmed milk instead of whole milk
Be sparing with butter, margarine, dripping, lard, oil, cream, cream cheese, fatty meat, pâté, mayonnaise, potato crisps and eat fried food only occasionally, using sunflower oil, corn oil, safflower oil or soya oil
It is a good idea to use polyunsaturated margarine and oils instead of butter, but remember to use it sparingly

Do not eat sugar or sugary foods
Sugar, glucose, jam, marmalade, honey, syrup, treacle, mincemeat, lemon curd, chocolate and sweets, cakes, pastries, sweet biscuits, sugar-coated breakfast cereals, all puddings made with sugar, tinned fruit in syrup, condensed milk, ordinary fruit squash, Ribena, sweet fizzy drinks, e.g. lemonade, Lucozade, Coca Cola

Eat less salt
Cut down on salt in cooking and at table

Watch your weight
The main aim is to have a normal body weight. If it starts creeping up, you must:
Cut down more on the fatty foods listed above.
Eat smaller portions of meat, fish, cheese and eggs
Limit yourself to 1 pint of skimmed milk or ½ pint of whole milk daily
Continue to eat your wholemeal bread, high-fibre cereals and vegetables

Food allowed freely
The following foods are very low in calories and you can fill up on these:
Fruit
Grapefruit, melon, rhubarb, gooseberries, loganberries, blackberries, lemon, red and black currants

Vegetables
Asparagus, aubergine, french and runner beans, bean sprouts, bamboo shoots, broccoli, brussel sprouts, courgetttes, cabbage, carrots, cauliflower, celeriac, chicory, celery, chives, chinese cabbage, cucumber, leeks, lettuce, marrow, mushrooms, mustard and cress, onions, peas, peppers, pumpkin, radishes, spinach, spring greens, swede, tomatoes, turnip, watercress

Condiments
Mustard, pepper, Worcester sauce, curry powder, vinegar, clear pickles, herbs and spices, tomato juice, clear soup (Bovril, Marmite, Oxo, soy sauce—remember these are high in salt)

Special diet products
These are an expensive and unncessary part of your diet. The items you may find useful, however, are:
Tablet and liquid saccharine sweeteners (avoid powdered sweeteners as they often contain sugar)
Sugar-free drinks, including Boots Diabetic Squash, Energen One-Cal drinks, Tab, Fresca, Diet Pepsi, Weight Watchers drinks and squash, PLJ (original and slightly sweetened), soda water, Vichy, Evian and Perrier water

Alcohol
Drink in moderation, i.e. an occasional glass of beer, dry sherry or wine. Avoid drinks with a high sugar content, such as sweet sherry and wine, port, liqueurs and sweet cider. There is no need to buy diabetic beer—ordinary beer is fine

CHAPTER 12
SMOKING

The World Health Organization has described tobacco-smoking as an epidemic. Indeed, as a cause of disease and death, smoking is today what the great epidemic diseases were in the past, and the 'contagion' is rapidly spreading to developing countries. In Britain about 100 000 deaths a year—a quarter of them under the age of 65—are caused by smoking. The average loss of life for someone smoking twenty cigarettes a day is 5 years and since about one in four smokers die prematurely as the result of smoking, the loss of life for an individual may be as much as 20 years. There are about 18 million smokers in Britain today and the average GP has about 600 patients on his list who smoke and about four deaths caused by smoking in his practice each year.

Smoking-related diseases

General

Since the early 1950s a number of studies have demonstrated the relationship between smoking and disease. Ninety per cent of the almost 40 000 deaths a year from lung cancer (the commonest form of cancer in men) in Britain are attributable to smoking, which also causes cancer of the larynx, oral cavity, oesophagus, pancreas and bladder. Doll and Peto* have estimated that 30% of all cancers are attributable to tobacco smoking.

It is also a major cause of cardiovascular disease, particularly coronary heart disease and peripheral arterial disease. It is estimated that 25% of deaths from coronary heart disease in men under the age of 65 are attributable to smoking and, because coronary heart disease is much commoner than lung cancer, the actual number of deaths from the former attributable to smoking is greater than the number of attributable deaths from lung cancer. Smoking is a particularly important factor in the younger age group and a man under 45 years who smokes twenty-five or more

*Doll, R. & Peto R. (1981) *The Causes of Cancer*. Oxford University Press, Oxford.

119

cigarettes a day may have a fifteen times greater risk of dying from a heart attack than if he were a non-smoker (Fig. 12.1).

Seventy five per cent of deaths from chronic bronchitis and emphysema are attributable to smoking and smoking also contributes to peptic ulceration.

Not only do smokers have a higher death rate than non-smokers, but they also suffer from more illness—for example, increased attacks of acute bronchitis—and it has been estimated that as many as 50 million working days are lost each year in Britain as a consequence of smoking.

Smokers consult their doctors more frequently than non-smokers and are higher users of hospital medical services.

However, the harmful effects of smoking are to some extent reversible. To stop smoking diminishes the excess risk from lung cancer, so that after 10–15 years it reverts almost to that of the life-long non-smoker (Fig. 12.2). The excess risk of death from

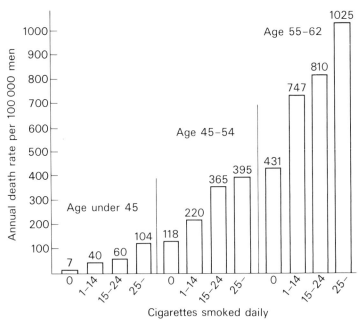

Fig. 12.1. Mortality rates from coronary heart disease of male smokers and non-smokers. (After Doll, R. & Peto, R. (1976) Mortality in relation to smoking: twenty years observations on male British doctors. *Brit. med. J.* **ii**, 1525–36.)

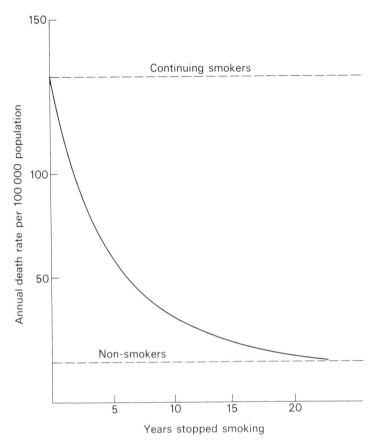

Fig. 12.2. Standardized death rate from lung cancer for cigarette smokers, ex-smokers for various lengths of time, and non-smokers. (After Doll, R. & Hill, A. B. (1964). Mortality in relation to smoking: ten years observations of British doctors. *Brit. med. J.* **i**, 1399.)

coronary heart disease, especially sudden death, is reduced more rapidly—by about 50% in the first year—and then gradually almost to that of the non-smoker by about 10 years.

Women
Women seem as susceptible to smoking-related diseases as men, but because of their relative delay in taking up smoking, the prevalence of the relevant diseases in women is still below that in

men, though rising. Moreover, smoking poses hazards peculiar to women: smoking during pregnancy retards fetal growth so that twice as many smokers as non-smokers give birth to premature babies and babies born to smokers have a higher perinatal mortality rate. There is also a greater risk of spontaneous abortion in smokers.

Smoking also increases the risks associated with taking combined oral contraceptive pills, especially in women over the age of 30 years. Older women on the pill who smoke thirty or more cigarettes daily have been shown to have a twenty times greater risk of coronary heart disease than those who never smoked.

Children

Children of mothers who smoke during pregnancy have been shown to be smaller and less intelligent than those of non-smokers and the risk of the infant developing a chest infection in the first year of life is doubled if parents smoke. Children of parents who smoke are more likely to smoke themselves, and smoking in children causes persistent and often productive coughing, increased chest infections and reduced ventilatory capacity.

Passive smoking

Recently, evidence has accumulated of the health risks to non-smokers of other people's smoking. Passive smoking causes impaired lung function and aggravates angina in sufferers, while young children are more likely to develop bronchitis if their parents smoke. In a study in Japan, the risk of lung cancer was significantly higher amongst non-smoking wives married to heavy smokers, than it was amongst those married to non-smokers.

Toxicity of tobacco

Tar products have for some time been known to have a carcinogenic effect, but the contribution which other noxious substances in tobacco smoke make to its disease effects are less certain. Carbon monoxide (which has an affinity for haemoglobin 245 times greater than that of oxygen) may be important in producing cardiovascular damage, and nicotine also has cardiovascular effects. Low-tar cigarettes are less damaging to the lungs than high-tar ones (and their introduction has contributed to the decline in lung cancer in men) but neither this change nor the switch from plain to filter cigarettes seems to have reduced the risk of coronary heart disease. Filter cigarettes are known to produce more carbon monoxide than plain ones.

Prevalence

Historical
In the 1950s roughly two-thirds of men and two-fifths of women smoked cigarettes. Since then smoking has fallen by 50% in men but remained much the same in women, so that there is now little difference between the two sexes (Fig. 12.3). The latest figures show that 42% of men and 37% of women are cigarette smokers but with the decline in the proportion of smokers there has been an increase in the consumption of those who do smoke by roughly 50% in men and 100% in women.

Social class
The decline in smoking is largely due to changes in the social-

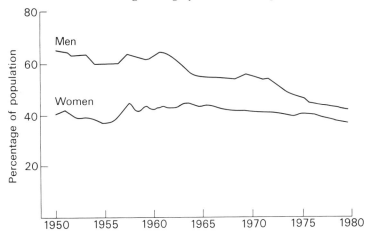

Fig. 12.3. Percentage of the adult population who are cigarette smokers in the U.K. from 1950 to 1980. (Sources: Tobacco Research Council Statistics of Smoking in the United Kingdom and Office of Population, Censuses and Surveys General Household Surveys.)

class pattern of the habit (Fig. 12.4). In 1960, smoking in men (about two-thirds of whom smoked) was more or less equally common in all social classes. By 1972 the proportion of social class V men who smoked was double that of social class I men, and now almost three times as many unskilled manual workers smoke as do professional men. Doctors have been particularly successful in stopping smoking: 80% are non-smokers (including 40% who are ex-smokers).

Cigarettes, pipes and cigars

Acknowledgement of the link between cigarette tar products and lung cancer has led to the introduction of filter-tipped cigarettes and subsequently cigarettes with a lower tar content. Nearly all cigarettes sold are now of the filter variety, and their average tar yield is only half of what it was 20 years ago. However, there is no such thing as a safe cigarette, merely perhaps a less dangerous one, and the cardiovascular risks associated with smoking do not appear to have been reduced by the introduction of low-tar filter cigarettes. Moreover, there is evidence that smokers compensate by smoking 'weaker' cigarettes more intensely.

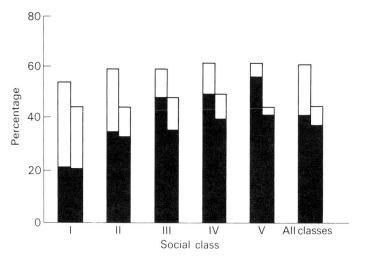

Fig. 12.4. Changes in the prevalence of smoking by social class from 1960 (□) to 1980 (■). Men are denoted by the left-hand column, women by the right-hand column. (Sources: Tobacco Research Council Statistics of Smoking in the United Kingdom and Office of Population, Censuses and Surveys General Household Surveys.)

Although pipe and cigar smoking appear less hazardous than cigarette smoking (the lung cancer risk being about one-quarter of that of cigarette smokers) those who switch from cigarettes to cigars or a pipe continue to inhale and thereby limit any possible 'benefit' resulting from such a change. Pipe and cigar smokers have about the same risk of developing cancer of the lip, mouth, larynx and oesophagus as do cigarette smokers.

Stopping smoking

Attitudes to smoking

Surveys show that about 70% of smokers want to stop smoking and that about the same proportion have, at some time or other, tried to do so. The majority of smokers also claim that they would stop if advised to do so by their doctors, but only a small proportion say that they have received such advice, though there is evidence that doctors do feel this an important task.

These findings are in spite of gross underestimation by the public of the harmful effects of smoking. Many are aware of the association between smoking and cancer, but only a few appear to know about the cardiovascular risks of smoking. Most think that the chances of dying in a road-traffic accident are greater than those of dying from smoking-related diseases, whereas road-traffic accident deaths in Britain each year are less than 10% of those due to smoking.

Nevertheless, large numbers of people have succeeded in stopping smoking and it is estimated that there are at least 8 million ex-smokers in Britain. The change in the social-class pattern of smoking (Fig. 12.4) is partly attributable to smoking cessation.

A number of factors in the social environment now favour smoking cessation. Surveys show that the majority of both smokers and non-smokers are in favour of further restrictions on smoking in public places including restaurants, there is pressure for the banning of advertising of cigarettes and increasing attention is given in the media to the smoking issue. However, related to average income, cigarettes are only one-third of the price they were 30 years ago.

Methods

Many approaches have been tried. These include techniques such as acupuncture, electro-aversive therapy, group therapy, hypnosis and a variety of drugs, including most recently nicotine chewing gum. All methods are undoubtedly effective for some individuals. But none, with the possible exception of nicotine chewing gum, has been shown to be more effective than another or than simple, firm advice from the patient's doctor.

Advice

The effectiveness of advice from the GP in helping patients to stop smoking has been demonstrated by recent research. In controlled trials, simple advice about stopping smoking given during normal consultations and reinforced with an anti-smoking leaflet and offer to see the patient again has been shown to result in sustained smoking cessation. It has been estimated that if more GPs adopted this procedure, half a million patients a year would stop smoking directly as a result of their doctors' advice. An appropriate leaflet to give to patients is the *Give Up Smoking (GUS) leaflet* (Fig. 12.5) available from the Health Education Council or Scottish Health Education Group.

Types of smoker

Cigarette smokers are by no means a homogenous group. There are different types of smoker: some, particularly the lighter smokers, may be able to stop without too much difficulty; others will be much more 'addicted'.

Someone who smokes twenty or more cigarettes a day should be considered a heavy smoker, but other guides to the dependence of the individual on smoking are how soon in the day the first cigarette is lit, and the previous experience of attempts to stop smoking.

Advice should not be specifically geared to patients with smoking-related diseases. However, advice to those who have already acquired such disease, although belated, is still very worthwhile and is likely to be even more effective, e.g. studies of the effectiveness of advice against smoking in patients who have had a myocardial infarction suggest that as many as two-thirds of those who smoke can be persuaded to stop. This compares with results showing that about one in five smokers are persuaded to

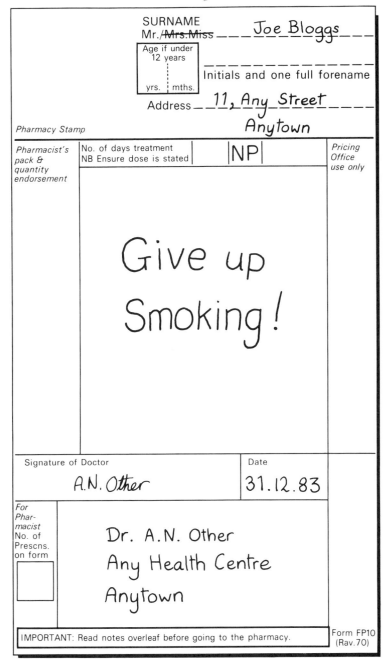

Fig. 12.5. GUS patient leaflet.

stop by advice from the doctor (and one in ten stop of their own volition).

Motivation and determination to stop are absolutely crucial. No smoker can stop unless he or she really wants to and efforts are unlikely to succeed if it is thought that stopping smoking is easy.

The basic features of advice on how to stop smoking are simple.

The first step is to record in the notes whether the patient is a smoker or not. Elicitation and recording of this information demonstrates to the patient the health significance of the habit. The recording (and the impact on the patient) may be facilitated by the use of sticky labels; some have used green or gold labels for non-smokers and red or black labels for smokers. The duration and quantity of smoking should also be recorded.

The reasons for giving up should be elicited from the patient, especially the positive ones. Remote hazards such as heart attacks, chronic bronchitis or even cancer in later life are unlikely to motivate the young smoker to stop. More significant will be personal factors like smell and 'bad breath', consideration for other people, especially children, and social pressures. Those already afflicted with smoking-related diseases are more likely to respond to the fear of further deterioration in their health and most can be honestly told that 'it is never too late' because, for example, although lung function will not improve after stopping smoking, further deterioration will be less rapid in the ex-smoker than in the continuing smoker.

A target date for stopping should be set. This should be some way ahead, preferably at a relatively stress-free time, such as holiday, or a time of changing routine. Motivation may be enhanced in the interim by regular review of the reasons for stopping, telling others about it and, better still, recruiting a fellow smoker, especially a spouse, to join in giving up. Switching to another brand, recording all cigarettes smoked in one day and when, where and why they are smoked, changing routine, avoiding tea or coffee and looking for alternatives to smoking, may all be found helpful in preparing to quit. Generally speaking, sudden complete withdrawal is more likely to succeed than gradual cutting down of the number of cigarettes smoked, but with some heavy smokers a period of cutting down may be the most effective technique. Conversely, some light or moderate smokers may be helped to stop smoking by the so-called 'saturation method' in which cessation is preceded by 1 or 2 days of smoking two or three times the normal number of cigarettes.

Some people find that offering themselves a reward is helpful, whether this is buying themselves a treat or merely saving (in a glass jar where they can see it) the money they would have spent on cigarettes. Advice is necessary on coping with difficulties after stopping. This includes the necessity to keep occupied, having something to nibble, chew or suck and something to occupy the hands. Danger times like tea-breaks and after meals or when having a drink need careful handling. Avoidance of others who smoke and of smoking environments at these times may be particularly crucial and the cooperation and support of friends and colleagues is vital. Support of a spouse is particularly important.

Tension and irritability cause particular problems and preparation to stop may well include learning techniques to cope with these. Relaxation exercises, taking deep breaths, yoga, etc., may all be found to be helpful in this respect, but regular physical exercise may be preferable for some. Follow-up of the patient by the doctor is important, to offer continuing help and support, as well as advice on managing difficulties. Vigilance is required for months and maybe years, and at least a year should elapse before a 'cure' is claimed. Most of those who finally succeed in stopping have tried and failed before, so initial failure by no means rules out eventual success.

A special problem which causes particular anxiety is that of weight gain. Although some smokers gain weight when they stop smoking, most do not, and most of those who do, revert to their normal weight after a period of time. It can be pointed out that to offset the health benefits gained by stopping smoking, the average smoker would have to increase his or her weight by 50%!

Nicotine chewing gum

Although the acquisition of the smoking habit is largely determined by social and psychological factors, there is evidence that dependence on the pharmacological effects of nicotine becomes a dominant influence for many, if not most, smokers. There has therefore been interest in providing an alternative source of nicotine, such as nicotine chewing gum as an aid to stopping smoking. Gum has the further advantage that it provides a substitute oral activity.

Several trials have shown that nicotine chewing gum may be more effective than other methods, particularly in smoking clinics, but its effectiveness in general practice needs to be more fully evaluated. Most studies to date have been conducted on highly selected smokers attending clinics which may not only include the more motivated smokers, but also the smokers who are more likely to be nicotine dependent. Moreover, other forms of treatment, such as group therapy or intensive support, are also included in the management of these patients.

The gum is currently available (on prescription only but not on the NHS) in two strengths: 2 mg and 4 mg. In using it, the manufacturers' instructions need to be carefully followed, in particular the advice that the gum should be chewed slowly and intermittently. The number of pieces needed daily varies with the individual, but the average is about ten. Experience to date indicates that no attempt should be made to reduce the use of the gum until the end of a 2- or 3-month period and that after that the amount should be slowly reduced. The majority of those who are able to stop smoking using the gum appear able to manage without it completely after a few months, but a small proportion seem to need to continue with it; but even in these people the hazards of nicotine chewing gum must be less than those of continuing smoking.

The exact role of nicotine chewing gum in the management of smoking cessation remains unclear, though it certainly seems to help some. It may have particular value in those who have tried and failed to stop simply with advice, and who, on the whole, will be the heaviest smokers who may be presumed to be more pharmacologically dependent on nicotine. On the other hand, by enabling the individual to cope with the social and psychological effects of stopping smoking without having, at the same time, to cope with the nicotine withdrawal, it may have a wide use. It should not be given to pregnant women or to children.

Prevention

A number of measures can be enforced which will prevent children starting and help smokers who wish to stop; these are summarized in the following checklist.

1 Ban on tobacco advertising and promotion.
2 Adequately funded health education.
3 Strong, changing health warnings on cigarette packets and such advertisements as remain.
4 (a) Regular, annual, significant tax increases.
(b) Differential taxation making higher tar cigarettes more expensive.
5 Increased provision for non-smokers in:
(a) public places;
(b) health premises;
(c) other places of work.
6 Ban on sale of cigarettes to children and young people

None of these measures will be effective in isolation: a comprehensive strategy embracing all these themes is necessary.

7 Establishment and progressive lowering of upper limits for emission products.
8 Assistance for those who require help in giving up smoking.
9 Collection of adequate information on smoking patterns and consequences to allow evaluation of these measures.

Summary of the doctor's role

1 Ask about and record in the patient's notes his/her smoking habits.
2 Seek an opportunity to inform a patient who smokes about the hazards of smoking and to offer advice in any consultation.
3 Give advice on how to stop and offer help and support.
4 Supplement such advice with appropriate literature, such as the GUS leaflet.
5 Consider the prescription of nicotine chewing gum.
6 Follow up the patient's attempts to stop smoking and encourage him or her to maintain their efforts.

More generally, the doctor should set a good example by not smoking himself/herself, prohibit smoking on practice premises, and support the medical profession's endorsement of the public desire for prohibition of all forms of tobacco promotion.

CHAPTER 13
ALCOHOL ABUSE

Two types of problem are caused by alcohol abuse.

Acute problems: drunkenness;
drinking and driving;
crime;
football hooliganism;
violence in the family.

Chronic problems: alcohol dependence;
physical disease, e.g. cirrhosis;
mental illness;
social problems, e.g. financial, marital, and
unemployment.

These overlap because many of the people who have acute problems either have, or go on to develop, chronic problems, particularly those who regularly have one or more on the acute list. For example, many of the people who have had more than one conviction for drunken driving also have chronic problems, so the acute problems listed above are not only difficulties in themselves: they may be symptoms of chronic problems. However, the two can be considered separately from the point of view of prevention.

Prevention of acute problems

Because the acute and chronic complications of alcohol abuse are so closely inter-related the prevention of both types of problems would best be achieved by the same solution—a more sensible use of alcohol. However, certain measures have been tried as a means of controlling the acute problems without attempting to tackle the basic problem (Table 13.1). The introduction of these types of steps only controls the acute manifestations of alcohol abuse. The real preventive measure would be to prevent alcohol abuse, thus preventing both acute and chronic problems.

Table 13.1. Attempted measures to control the acute problems related to alcohol.

Attempted solution	Effect
Drunkenness Because it was felt that drunkenness in Scotland was due, at least in part, to the pressure to drink quickly in the limited hours the pubs were open, the licensing laws were changed and pubs are now open much longer hours.	This measure has only been in operation a few years but it does seem that the problem of drunkenness has been reduced.
Football hooliganism Prohibition of the sale of alcohol in football stadia. Refusal of entry to people who are drunk or who are carrying alcohol.	These measures have been effective.
Drunken driving Introduction of the breathalyser. Publicity informing motorists that campaigns against drunken driving will be mounted at times of high prevalence, e.g. around Christmas time. Tightening up of legal loopholes to ensure that the person who is detected with high levels of alcohol in his bloodstream will actually be convicted, no matter how clever his barrister may be. Gaoling of offenders	The introduction of the breathalyser in 1967 was followed by a marked decline in the proportion of deaths on the road caused by alcohol. However, the proportion has risen steadily since then, suggesting that drivers have become less worried by the risks of detection and conviction.
Violence in the family The provision of 'battered wives hostels'. The granting of legal injunctions to women being assaulted by ex-husbands.	Of limited effectiveness in terms of the total number of women and children at risk but these measures are effective for the small number of women who make use of them.

Prevention of chronic problems

The extent of the problem is difficult to assess, not only because different people use different definitions of alcoholism and because the drinker himself may conceal his problem. However, on the basis of a number of different surveys it has been suggested that one in twenty-five of the population in England and Wales, and one in ten of the population of Scotland and Northern

Ireland is harmed by the effects of alcohol, either on themselves or on another member of their family. One indicator of the incidence of alcoholism that is often used as a measure of the prevalence of alcoholism is the death rate from cirrhosis and this has been increasing in recent years, suggesting that the problems are increasing (Fig. 13.1). It appears that the increase is particularly marked among women and younger people.

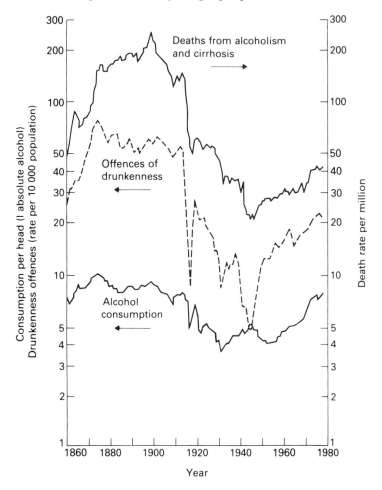

Fig. 13.1. Deaths from alcoholism and cirrhosis, offences of drunkenness and consumption of alcohol (U.K.) in England and Wales 1860–1978. (Office of Health Economics (1981) *Alcohol: Reducing the Harm.* OHE, London.)

The causes of alcohol abuse may be divided into two types: social and personal. The social causes determine how many people in a society are affected, the personal causes determine which particular individuals in that society are more likely to be affected.

Social causes
The level of consumption
Ledermann, a French demographer, advanced a theory in 1956 which continues to be the centre of controversy. Previously it had been thought that there were two distinct populations of alcohol consumers—those who were alcoholics and those who were not —and that the two populations were unrelated. It was believed that the number of people who were heavy consumers and who suffered from the effects of alcohol abuse bore no relationship to the numbers of people who were consuming alcohol without harmful effects, e.g. it was believed that it was possible to have a high average level of consumption in a community with a low prevalence of problems, and Italy was cited as an example of such a country. In statistical terms a bimodal distribution was believed to obtain with two distinct populations of drinkers (Fig. 13.2). As a consequence of this it was believed that measures to prevent alcoholism should concentrate on the small proportion of heavy drinkers and that measures to control the total amount of alcohol consumed by a society were irrelevant.

However, Ledermann proposed that the distribution was unimodal and that an increase in the total amount of alcohol consumed in society would be followed by an increase in the number of problems as the curve, which is a lognormal curve, was shifted to the right (Fig. 13.3).

As one would expect, the position is not as clear-cut as this and patterns of alcohol consumption vary from one community to another. Most people interested in the prevention of alcohol abuse, however, now believe that measures to control the total amount of alcohol consumed in society play a part in preventing alcoholism, i.e. they support the Ledermann hypothesis, which the alcohol industry, not surprisingly, does not. The historical evidence supports the hypothesis that the numbers of people

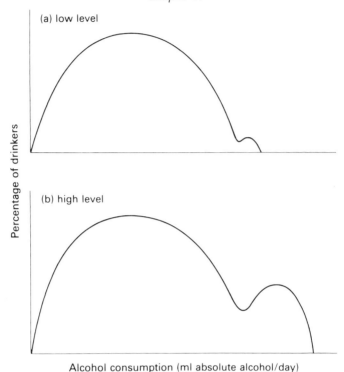

Fig. 13.2. Alcohol consumption patterns in two countries with (a) a low and (b) a high level of problems, based on the bimodal theory.

suffering from the effects of alcohol abuse is a function of the total amount of alcohol consumed although no one would argue that this was the only causal factor.

Consumption can be controlled by the measures outlined in Table 13.2, but the opposition to such moves is powerful and has political 'clout'.

Social attitudes

Certain social attitudes also influence the number of people affected by alcohol abuse (Table 13.3). Such social attitudes are important. They also change in the course of time but it is difficult to influence such attitudes by health education or public-information campaigns. There is, however, evidence to suggest that health education campaigns have reduced the pressure on

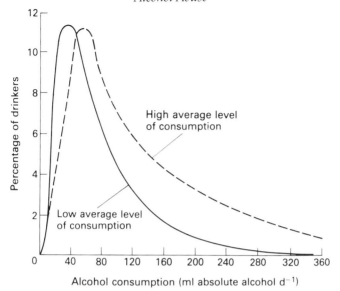

Fig. 13.3. Alcohol consumption patterns based on the unimodal Ledermann hypothesis in countries with low and high levels of consumption.

drivers who prefer not to drink: fewer hosts and 'friends' now press the driver to have 'one for the road'.

Personal causes

Social factors determine the number of people adversely affected in a society. Personal factors determine which particular members of that society are more likely to be affected. Two types of personal factors can be identified: (i) the individual's personality; (ii) the strain upon him. The more resilient and stable the person, the less likely is he to become dependent on alcohol: the greater the strain, the more likely is he to become dependent and these two factors are obviously inter-related. The more stable and resilient the individual, the better able is he to cope with personal disasters such as redundancy, divorce or bereavement. Conversely, the person who does not have such a strong personality may become dependent on alcohol simply because he needs the effects of alcohol to help him cope with the challenges of ordinary social life, such as going to dances and parties or minor disappointments and set-backs at work.

Table 13.2. Possible measures for reducing alcohol consumption

Measure	Mechanism	Obstacles
Increase in price		
The price of alcohol relative to the average income has declined by 50% in the U.K. between 1949 and 1979	Chancellor of Exchequer's decision to increase tax	Opposition of alcohol industry Effect on Retail Price Index in which alcohol is included
Advertising controls		
Advertising is said by industry only to affect 'brand loyalty' but it also influences social attitudes	Imposition of legal controls on advertising. These could be introduced by a Secretary of State for Health, if he were dissatisfied with the effects of present voluntary controls	Opposition of advertising industry
Controls on availability		
Alcohol has become more easily available, especially for women shopping in supermarkets	Control of number of licensed premises by magistrates	Opposition by retail trade

Preventive strategies

Primary prevention

This requires a combination of educational and social measures. Education about alcohol should not be presented in isolation but in the context of a general health-education programme, and the objectives have to be very simple in order to influence individual attitudes and beliefs.

1 To give insight into the reasons why people drink alcohol in the way they do.

2 To teach people about the relative strength of different drinks.

3 To give information on the early warning signs of alcoholic dependence.

4 To help people to be able to analyse advertisements.

In addition to these objectives a comprehensive health-education programme also attempts to change social beliefs and attitudes.

Table 13.3. Relevant attitudes

Relevance of attitudes	Evidence
Drunkenness	
Tolerant attitudes promote heavy consumption	Drunkenness is condoned in certain cultures, e.g. the Scottish, to a greater degree than in others, e.g. the Jewish
Abstinence	
Intolerance towards abstinence increases the number of people drinking and driving.	Intolerance appears to be decreasing and it also appears that the intro-
If abstinence is regarded as abnormal, alcohol consumption will be re- garded as normal and total con- sumption will increase	duction of non-alcoholic drinks to business lunches, with a reduction in the pressure to drink, is taking place and is generally welcomed
Intolerance is particularly pronounced in certain social situations, such as business lunches	

Educational initiatives have to be complemented by environmental measures, i.e. those affecting the environment in which
the individual makes his decisions, such as price increases and
the control of advertising.

Secondary prevention

People do not become dependent on alcohol overnight; the process is a gradual one which follows a typical order of occurrence
as listed below. (After Chick, J. & Duffy, D. C. (1980) The
developmental ordering of symptoms in the alcohol dependence
syndrome. In *Aspects of Alcohol and Drug Dependence* (eds
Maddon, J. S., Walker, R. & Kenyon, W. H.) Pitman, London.)

> Completely unable to keep to a drink limit
> Need more than companions (e.g. going for
> drink between rounds)
> Difficulty preventing getting drunk
> Spending more time drinking
> Missing meals drinking
> Black-outs, memory loss
> Giving up interests because drinking interferes
> Restless without a drink

Change to drinking same on working days as on
days off
Organizing day to ensure supply
Change to drinking same amounts whatever
mood
Passing out while drinking in public
Trembling after drinking the day before
Times when cannot think of anything but getting
a drink
Morning retching or vomiting
Sweating excessively at night
Withdrawal fit
Morning drinking
Decreased tolerance to alcohol
Waking up panicking or frightened
Hallucinations

Secondary prevention, therefore, depends on the recognition of this trend when a person asks for advice about his drinking, or, much more commonly, when his abuse of alcohol is the cause of a problem which brings him into contact with professional services. When a drunken-driving offence, the symptoms of gastritis, a road-traffic accident or difficulties at work brings the person who is developing dependence on alcohol into contact with his GP, another doctor, a probation officer, his personnel manager or another source of professional help an opportunity for secondary prevention is offered. The professional must:
1 be aware of the possibility of alcohol abuse;
2 be able to ask the right questions;
3 know how to counsel the person himself or have access to a counselling service.
The key to effective secondary prevention is, therefore, appropriate professional education.

Relevant agencies

In many parts of the country local Councils on Alcoholism do much to educate the public and to co-ordinate services. They are supported by Alcohol Concern, a national agency on alcohol misuse and AAA (Action Against Alcohol Abuse), a political pressure group.

CHAPTER 14
ACCIDENTS

The earliest definition of the word 'accident', the Middle English definition, is that it is 'an unforeseen contingency', and it was only later, in 1490, that the meaning of 'chance' or 'fortune' was introduced. It is the latter meaning that many people now associate with the term. Accidents are believed to occur because of 'bad luck' and, in consequence, the potential for prevention is not considered to be as great as it is for other problems such as heart disease or cancer. The common causes of accidental death are shown in Fig. 14.1.

Road-traffic accidents

The epidemiological data reveal important facts about road-traffic accidents.

1 They are more common in males than females.

2 Among motor-vehicle users the peak mortality occurs in the age range 15–24 years.

3 The motor cycle is the most dangerous form of transport.

4 Among pedal-cycle users the peak mortality occurs in the age range 10–14 years.

5 Pedestrian mortality is highest in childhood and old age.

6 Alcohol plays a very important part in the causation of road-traffic accidents.

Studies of road-traffic accidents reveal that most are caused by the behaviour of the person involved; the low proportion of accidents caused by illness is due not to the unimportance of illness as a potential causal factor but to the stringent regulations governing people with disabilities who wish to drive.

The strategy for prevention has four main elements:

1 Changes in the physical environment, e.g. improved car design, legal requirements to maintain cars in a safe condition, e.g. the MOT test and the regulations specifying the condition of

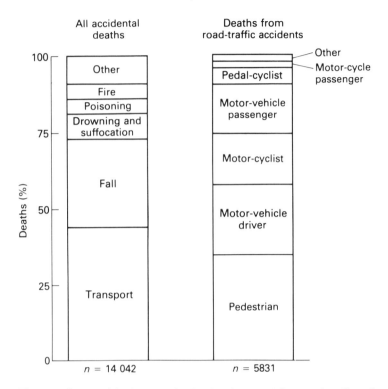

Fig. 14.1. Causes of deaths in England and Wales in 1980 from road-traffic and other accidents. (After Donaldson R. J. & Donaldson, L. J. (1983) *Essential Community Medicine* MTP, Lancaster.)

car tyres; new road building and the alteration of accident black spots.

2 Changes in the social environment, e.g. changing attitudes to drinking and driving; the introduction of the breathalyser; seat-belt legislation; sanctions approved by society to control the behaviour of those who endanger others, e.g. the penalties for reckless driving and the restrictions on the use of high-powered motor cycles.

3 Personal preventive services, e.g. the advice given to people with disabilities by their doctors and by the Medical Advisory Branch of the Driver and Vehicle Licensing Centre; the driving test.

4 Education, e.g. education of parents of young children about

road safety and the need for restraints in cars; education of young children, e.g. the Green Cross Code; education of young motor-cyclists through the STEP (Schools Transport Education Programme) training-scheme courses for those over school-leaving age; publicity campaigns about drinking and driving; the driving test requiring people to learn how to drive in schools of motoring; education of old people about safe road use.

There is therefore no simple means of preventing road-traffic accidents. An integrated policy is required. Responsibility rests principally with the County Councils and District Councils responsible for both highway maintenance and road-safety education.

Home accidents

These are most common at the two ends of life—childhood (see p. 55–73) and old age. The commonest types of fatal accident in old age are falls and fires.

Falls
A number of different factors contribute to the increased incidence of falls in old age.
1 Disorders of balance which may be the side-effects of prescribed medication, such as anti-hypertensive medication or tranquillizers.
2 Locomotor disorders which increase the probability of tripping.
3 Cardiovascular disorders resulting in drop attacks.
4 Visual impairment.
5 A home environment with uneven floors, unlighted steps and stairs and loose wires.
Good medical care is therefore at least as important in the prevention of falls as the provision of safe environment.

Fires
The most common cause of fires at all ages are cigarettes and matches and this remains so in old age. The other common causes are unsafe heating apparatus, cooking appliances and electric blankets. In old age the presence of dementia, visual impairment

and disabling disease which impairs mobility all increase the risk of fire. Thus, the prevention of fire requires:

1 the prevention of cigarette smoking;

2 the encouragement of the use of cigarette lighters rather than matches;

3 the provision of housing with safe heating and cooking appliances.

In addition, the installation of fire alarms in hotels and institutions is of importance. The supervision of this work is undertaken by fire prevention officers of Fire Services, who are in turn supervized by the Home Office.

CHAPTER 15
ENVIRONMENTAL THREATS TO HEALTH

In developed countries relatively few people now die or become disabled as a result of the physical environment in which they live. The great environmental problems of the nineteenth century —smokey air and polluted water—have been overcome and it is the social environment in which people live and their life-style that now cause many more deaths than the physical environment. This does not mean that there are no health hazards in the physical environment or that we can relax our efforts to keep the environment safe. Indeed, the opposite is the case. The environment has become, and remains, relatively safe because there is a set of laws to protect it and because there are groups of professionals dedicated to environmental protection. We must become increasingly vigilant as the number of potential hazards to the environment grows each year.

Outstanding environmental issues

The many problems in the physical environment can be classified under six principal headings.

Radiation
This includes the threat of nuclear war, the greatest potential threat to human health. The health hazards of radiation are now a major source of public concern. The leak at Three Mile Island, the concern about Windscale, the opposition to the dumping of radioactive waste under ground or under the sea, have all received prominent publicity, fostered by the activities of groups such as Greenpeace. This growth in public interest has been reflected and expressed in the growing political influence of the environmental lobby, most notably by the success of the Green Party in West Germany.

Air pollution
Particulate pollution—fog—is no longer a major problem but pollution with sulphur dioxide, the cause of 'acid rain' and exhaust emission, the cause of smog, are steadily increasing problems.

Water pollution
Industrial toxic waste and nitrates from fertilizers are the two main pollutants. Both rivers and the seas are at risk.

Noise
This is now the commonest cause of complaints to environmental health departments.

Food pollution
This may take place during production, e.g. by the addition of colouring and preservatives, or during distribution and cooking. Food poisoning remains a major health problem.

Housing problems
The old problems—overcrowding, homelessness and unsatisfactory dwellings—still persist, with additional problems resulting from high-rise flats and the large estates created in an attempt to solve the traditional problems quickly. These new environments have spawned new problems.

Preventing environmental hazards

The prevention of environmental health problems requires two approaches: the control of known hazards and the prevention of new hazards.

The control of known hazards
A large number of hazards are known and there are a range of laws and regulations to control them. Some are general laws covering the whole field of public health, e.g. the Public Health Act 1961, the Health Service and Public Health Act 1968, and the Food and Drugs Act 1955. Others are much more specific, e.g. the

Liquid Egg Pasteurization Regulation 1963 and the Slaughter-house (Hygiene) Regulations 1977. However, laws and regulations do not prevent problems by themselves. They have to be enforced and a number of different services are responsible for enforcement. Among the most important are:

1 The Health and Safety Executive which is responsible for occupational health with the Employment Medical Advisory Service as its medical arm.

2 Veterinary surgeons and scientific officers of the Ministry of Agriculture, Fisheries and Food.

3 The National Radiological Protection Board.

4 The Public Health Laboratory Service which acts as a centre of expertise and information on communicable diseases.

5 The Regional Water Authorities.

6 Staff at the Department of Health and Social Security.

7 Environmental Health Officers.

8 Medical Officers of Environmental Health.

The list of people involved is impressive but the number of different services can create problems, since responsibility for certain environmental problems is shared by a number of different services and by a number of different government departments, e.g. the Department of Health is responsible for medical advice on health hazards but is not responsible for the control of all environmental health hazards.

The style of control

Although there are laws and regulations with specific sanctions, the control of known hazards depends at least as much on education of those who have the power to cause or control the hazard as on the threat of punishment. In seeking to control industry, Government seeks an approach based on cooperation not conflict. This means that it must recognize the problems of industry, notably the cost of pollution control and the time needed for an industry to introduce new standards of pollution control, when introducing new legislation. Similarly, environmental health officers do not simply threaten shopkeepers and restauranteurs with fines and imprisonment. The sanctions for those who breach the food hygiene regulations are used from time to time, but the environmental health officers spend a higher proportion of their time educating those who are handling food and helping them to improve their standards and skills than they spend in the courts. They are primarily health educators, not health policemen.

Preventing new hazards

The control of known hazards is difficult; the detection of new hazards even more so. Each year a larger number of new chemical compounds are developed by industry and as biotechnology becomes more widespread a new potential source of hazards has to be kept under surveillance.

Some chemicals that will be used as drugs or food additives obviously receive close scrutiny but the many other chemicals that are produced for other purposes may also constitute health hazards. It is, therefore, essential to maintain strict controls over the introduction of new drugs or new food additives and to have systems for detecting hazards caused by other chemicals. Cancer registration is one such system; the detection of an increase in the incidence of one particular type of cancer and its association with a particular occupational group allows the identification of carcinogens, although the time taken for cancers to reach a symptomatic stage is such that it is difficult for cancer registration to detect new carcinogens quickly.

Obstacles to environmental health

In some instances, industry actively campaigns against the introduction of measures to reduce or prevent environmental health hazards. More commonly, the reason why change does not come about more quickly is simply that there is inertia in any political and bureaucratic system and action is not taken until sufficient pressure has built up to move the system. This is perfectly illustrated in the history of the legislation to control the dumping of toxic solid waste—'fly-tipping'.

The making of law

The following sequence of events indicates the difference between scientific evidence and public pressure as motivating forces behind a change in the law.

1963 Death of sheep in south-east England as a result of dumping rusty cans of pesticide.

Government appoints the Technical Committee on the Disposal of Toxic Solid Wastes.

1970 Committee publishes report after twenty meetings in 6 years.

Royal Commission on Environmental Pollution appointed: the commissioners decide to investigate 'fly-tipping'.

1971 Royal Commission presses Minister for action: no action taken.

1972 Lorry driver Lonnie Downes reports to the Conservation Society that he has been threatened with dismissal after refusing to dump toxic solid waste.

Conservation Society informs press: Birmingham *Sunday Mercury* prints scoop on 10 January.

Parliament debates issue: Minister maintains that legislation is impossible before 1974.

24 February: 36 t of cyanide are discovered on a children's playground in Nuneaton: press and media launch attack on Government.

8 March: Bill to control dumping of toxic solid waste has first reading.

20 March: Bill becomes law.

As was reported in *The Times* Editorial of 7 March, 1972, 'It is instructive to note what did and what did not prompt the Government to squeeze a Bill as a matter of urgency into an already crowded legislative programme. The urgent representations of an official commission composed of distinguished persons who were moved by 'the disturbing cases which have come to our knowledge of local problems and anxieties' did not. Headlines about drums of cyanide waste on derelict land in the Midlands did.'

This case study, described by Lord Ashby in his brilliant and entertaining book *Reconciling Man with the Environment*, illustrates the politics of prevention perfectly. Health hazards, although of vital importance both to the public health and those who specialize in their control, do not necessarily have the same degree of priority for politicians and they have to be moved up the agenda before action will be taken.

COMMON HEALTH PROBLEMS

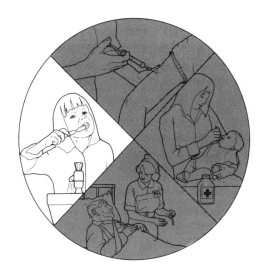

CHAPTER 16
PREVENTION OF MENTAL ILLNESS

Mental illness is responsible for the use of 31% of all hospital beds and is a very common cause of disability and handicap. However, its prevention is difficult, not only because the causes of mental illness are not fully understood but also because there is disagreement on its nature and definition: some people regard even the term 'mental illness' as misleading. Without being drawn into this complicated and heated debate two types of problem can be identified, which are not, however, clearly distinguished from one another.

1 Those that are qualitatively different from the normal range of thinking, i.e. schizophrenia and the psychological sequelae of dementia. These disorders are largely responsible for the hospital admissions.

2 Those that are qualitatively similar to the normal range of thinking and feeling, i.e. emotional disorders, anxiety and depression. These disorders are largely responsible for the high rates of prescribing of psychotropic drugs by GPs.

There is an overlap between the two types of disorder because severe depression may be a disorder with a biochemical cause, qualitatively different from the normal range of depressive moods.

Prevention of schizophrenia

Primary
The cause of schizophrenia is unknown so there is no scope for primary prevention.

Secondary
GPs may not diagnose schizophrenia when the symptoms are first presented. Early detection can improve the long-term prognosis if the person's symptoms can be controlled and family breakdown prevented but there is no case for screening for schizophrenia.

Chapter 16

Tertiary

This is the most important aspect of prevention. It has two main objectives which are closely related:
1 prevention of family breakdown;
2 prevention of long-term hospitalization.

Tertiary prevention requires the range of services listed in Table 16.1.

Prevention of dementia

Primary

The majority of elderly people affected by dementia are affected by Alzheimer's disease, or senile dementia of Alzheimer's type (SDAT) as it is sometimes called. The cause of this disease is not

Table 16.1. Tertiary prevention in schizophrenia

Service	Service implications
Control of symptoms by appropriate use of phenothiazine tranquillizers	Adequate training of GPs Use of community psychiatric nursing services to link hospital services with community services Easy access to skilled psychiatric advice for diagnosis and planning of treatment
Long-term surveillance and support	Need for good liaison between hospital and community services Need for well organized record system
Support and stimulation for the sufferer	Appropriate training of all professionals who come in contact with sufferers Provision of day-hospital facilities with supervised workshops and occupational-therapy departments
Support for relatives	Adequate time must be given to support relatives by psychiatric community nurses, GPs and social workers Relatives need relief by offering the sufferer day-hospital attendance or by admission of the affected person to hospital from time to time
Group homes for those who have no family or whose family support has disintegrated	Provision of a range of different types of group home

known and it is therefore not preventable. The minority of cases are due to atherosclerotic or multi-infarct dementia, i.e. to a number of small strokes. Although there is now evidence that atherosclerosis is preventable there is, as yet, no evidence that the measures that are known to prevent the effects of atherosclerosis in the heart and arteries of the lower limbs are also effective in the prevention of multi-infarct dementia.

The treatment of high blood pressure in old age is one aspect of the prevention of arterial disease that is particularly relevant because it is known its reduction reduces the risk of a stroke. There is, however, no evidence that blood pressure reduction reduces the risk of suffering the type of small stroke that is the cause of multi-infarct dementia; and there is concern that reduction of the levels of blood pressure in an older person may reduce the perfusion of the brain to a level at which the brain tissue is threatened by lack of oxygen. Multi-infarct dementia must therefore be regarded as neither preventable not treatable at the present time.

A very small proportion of people who are referred because other people have noticed that they have slowly become more confused have brain diseases that are treatable but there is little scope for primary prevention (Table 16.2).

Secondary
There are certain complications of dementia which increase the degree of confusion but are, in fact, avoidable.
1 Negative attitudes towards the person with dementia.
2 Isolation.

Table 16.2. Common treatable causes of brain failure

More common treatable causes of brain disease	Scope for primary prevention
Myxoedema	None, but early detection is important
Vitamin B_{12} deficiency	None, but early detection is important
Alcohol abuse	Counselling and support of the elderly person at times of crisis
Normal pressure hydrocephalus	None, but early detection is important

3 Sensory deprivation due to unreported visual failure or hearing loss.

4 Unreported physical illness.

5 Mistakes with prescribed medication.

6 Unreported depression.

7 Family tension: this both causes intellectual deterioration and is created by it.

The early detection of these treatable causes is important but there is no evidence that all elderly people should be screened for these conditions.

Because the two main causes of dementia—Alzheimer's disease and multiple infarcts—are untreatable there would seem to be little possibility of benefit from early detection of people suffering from dementia, but this is not the case. Benefit is achieved not by affecting the progress of dementia but by preventing the harmful effects that can occur from the complications

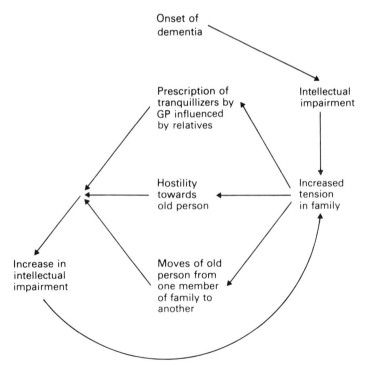

Fig. 16.1. Cycles of deterioration

of dementia. Early detection of families who are having problems coping with an elderly person suffering from dementia is particularly important because family tension can aggravate the elderly person's intellectual impairment. It is also important because the probability of admission of an old person with dementia to hospital is influenced at least as much by the anxiety of other people as by the degree of his or her intellectual impairment (Fig. 16.1). If the primary-care team runs a surveillance programme, making contact with those elderly people who

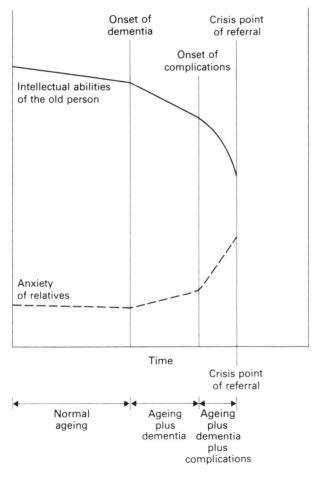

Fig. 16.2. Natural progression of dementia in an old person living with relatives.

have not made contact with any members of the team in the course of the previous year, some cases in which these complications are starting to have an effect will be detected and steps can be taken to reduce the risk of a crisis and hospitalization (Fig. 16.2. and 16.3).

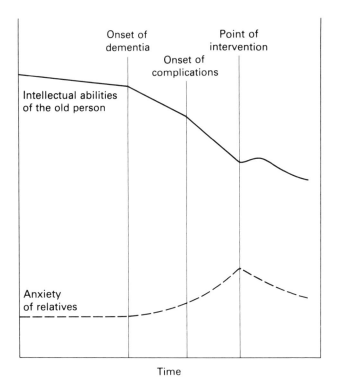

Fig. 16.3. Effects of early intervention; probably when the problem is detected in the course of consultation on another matter.

Tertiary
The tertiary prevention of dementia requires the prevention of the complications listed in Table 16.3 or the mitigation of their effects where they cannot be prevented.

Prevention of emotional disorders

In the past, cases of depression were divided into two types: endogenous and reactive. The former was considered to be qualitatively different from the depressed feelings that everyone experiences from time to time, being due to some internal biochemical cause; whereas the latter was simply a more severe degree of the type of depressed feelings that are universally experienced. In recent years, the two types of disorder have not been so clearly demarcated from one another, although it is still thought that there is a type of depression caused by a biochemical disorder. Research into the biochemical and neuropharmacological causes of depression continues but no cause has been found, so the main scope lies in the prevention of depression that is simply a more severe degree of the type of feeling we all experience.

There is no evidence that any of the people suffering from anxiety are suffering from a specific biochemical disorder; people who suffer from anxiety are suffering from a reaction, like most of those people who seek help for depression. Three inter-related factors can be identified in the causation of anxiety and depression.

1 Individual personality.
2 Individual environment.
3 The amount and quality of support received from close friends and family at times of crisis or during periods of pressure.

Prevention by influencing personality traits
The psychological characteristics of an individual determine the likelihood that he will become anxious or depressed in certain circumstances. It is very difficult for doctors, nurses or teachers to influence a person's personality, and thereby reduce the risk of anxiety and depression, because the main influence is his family. However, attempts are made to help parents bring up their children in a family culture in which the child is given an opportunity to express his emotions honestly and easily, and to

Table 16.3.

Effect of complication on intellectual function	Scope for professional action	Scope for community action
Isolation Isolation has been shown in research on brainwashing to cause disorientation, paranoid depression and what may be called a disintegration of the personality	Try to arrange: more trips out of the home more visitors into the home more stimulation in the home by provision of a pet or a television.	Support for voluntary organizations trying to develop day centres and home-visiting schemes. Development of transport schemes.
Sensory deprivation Sensory deprivation has been shown to produce disorientation and paranoid thoughts in young, fit volunteers. Many elderly people with dementia also have deafness or visual failure. Those with severe degrees of dementia are unable to report their problem and seek help.	Awareness of dangers of deafness and blindness for someone with dementia. Exclusion of deafness caused by wax in ears by looking in ears when examining older people. Be able to check batteries on hearing aids. Be able and prepared to instruct relatives and friends of a person with hearing loss how best to communicate with the person. Check that the person with dementia has, and uses, their glasses.	Development of services for elderly people with hearing failure and visual failure. Support for voluntary organizations.
Family tensions Hostility towards the old person, or towards other relatives, and frequent moves of the old person increases the confusion	Discuss with relatives their reaction to the dementia and to the burden they have to bear; encourage them to admit hostile feelings or resentment by telling them that, in virtually every family caring for an old person with dementia, these feelings occur from time to time. Be able to give the relatives advice on the financial benefits available. Enquire about the old person and the care the relatives are giving her whenever one of	Development of relief services such as day centres, day hospitals and the regular admission of the old person to hospital from time to time.

	Be prepared to try to achieve the admission of the old person to a long-stay bed or an old people's home if the strain has become too great for the relatives.	
Unreported physical illness Elderly people with dementia are: more likely to develop an acute confusional reaction to physical illness; less able to describe physical symptoms or to refer themselves to the doctor. In addition, relatives may ascribe other deterioration in intellectual function to their dementia.	Educate relatives and helpers that deterioration in intellectual function which occurs in the course of a few days or weeks should be suspected as being due to a disease other than dementia, and referred to the doctor.	Develop educational services for the relatives and helpers of elderly people with dementia.
Adverse reaction to drugs Elderly people with dementia are: more sensitive to certain drugs; less able to report side-effects; more likely to make mistakes;	Prescribe: as little as possible; in as small a dose as possible; in as simple a regime as possible; with adequate instruction and advice.	Improve professional education about drug problems in old age and about the steps that can be taken to reduce the risk of mistakes made by the old person.
Negative social attitudes and depression When the diagnosis is made the person is in danger of being labelled 'a dement' and some people have low expectations of, and negative attitudes towards, dements; they: never correct them if a mistake is made; never inform them if their behaviour is upsetting others; never include them in any serious discussion; always refer to them as 'being like babies' and treat them as such; assume that people with dementia have no feelings.	Educate younger people that someone with dementia still has a mind and can still feel anxious and depressed. Encourage younger people to correct a person with dementia who makes mistakes and behaves badly. Teach younger people how to provide stimulation for a person with dementia, e.g. by reminding them of the date and discussing current events.	Education of public and professionals.

develop a stable framework of values that will allow him to make decisions when faced with difficult choices. Obviously it is extremely difficult to achieve this but the following measures are tried:

1 Parentcraft education for teenage children in school, for prospective parents in antenatal classes and for parents at home through the visits of the health visitor.

2 The provision of services for people whose marriages are in difficulty to help them sort out their difficulties, if necessary by divorce, without doing too much damage to the children in the process. This is undertaken by GPs, social workers, health visitors and marriage-guidance counsellors.

3 The provision of a caring, stable environment in school for those whose homes are very unstable or uncaring.

Although these approaches have had some effect the scope for prevention of emotional disorders by modifying personality traits is limited.

Prevention by environmental engineering

The environmental factors that put people under stress and lead to either anxiety or depression, depending upon the person's personality and the support he is receiving, may be divided into two types: chronic problems and life crises, although they are obviously interrelated. It is, however, more appropriate to think of these as two types of environmental factors rather than using the imprecise term 'stress'.

Common chronic problems contributing to emotional disorders include:

> an unhappy family life;
> an unhappy marriage;
> poverty;
> bad housing;
> living in an environment in which crime and
>   vandalism are common;
> isolation;
> being a single parent;
> unemployment;
> chronic physical disease.

Common acute crises contributing to emotional disorders are:

divorce;	bankruptcy;
bereavement;	the onset of disease;
redundancy;	eviction.

Life crises are difficult to prevent and efforts have therefore to be directed at improving the support for someone coping with such crises. The chronic social problems that cause anxiety and depression are, in part, preventable, although there is little that a doctor, nurse or social worker can do on his own to solve the nation's housing problem or to prevent poverty. The main contribution a doctor or nurse can make is to help the individual cope with problems and to help him find ways of overcoming them, e.g. by helping solve his marital problems or helping him obtain rehousing.

Prevention by strengthening the support system

The probability that a person will become anxious or depressed depends upon the support that he is given by people who are close to him. The person who has a stable, happy marriage and who lives near his relatives with whom he has a close and happy relationship is less likely to become anxious or depressed than the person who lives alone or in an unhappy marriage, far from friends and family. It is obviously impossible for professional workers to provide support of the amount or quality that is given by a loving family to someone who is isolated and vulnerable. However, professionals can help by providing support for people living under the stress of chronic social problems or who are coping with the consequences of an acute crisis. Examples of this are the support given by:

1 a health visitor to a single parent looking after two small children.

2 a social worker to a woman who is trying to divorce a violent husband.

3 a GP to someone recently widowed.

In addition to this type of professional support, self-help groups, which have grown in number and strength in recent years, play a very important part in the prevention of anxiety and depression. Some people find the support of those with practical experience of their problem of greater help than the advice of a professional who, no matter how expert he may be, has not had to face a similar problem or crisis.

CHAPTER 17
PREVENTION OF OCCUPATIONAL DISEASE

It was once believed that the loss of work due to sickness absence was a valid indicator of the state of health of the nation because it was thought that the number of days lost was directly proportional to the level of disease in the community. However, the more closely sickness absence has been studied, the less valid do its rates appear to be as indicators of the prevalence of disease. Disease prevalence is obviously an important factor determining absence rates, but it is only one factor among many (Table 17.1).

The importance of the social factors influencing sickness absence is illustrated by the fact that sickness absence rates are rising in most developed countries (Table 17.2) although there is no evidence that the incidence or prevalence of disabling diseases have risen.

The medical conditions responsible for sickness absence are shown in Table 17.3. The causes differ between men and women; women lose a higher percentage of days due to neuroses and ill-defined conditions such as 'debility'. Men lose proportionately more due to respiratory and circulatory disorders. One notable

Table 17.1. Some factors known to influence sickness absence. (After Taylor, P. J. (1979) Aspects of sickness absence. In *Current Approaches to Occupational Medicine*, ed. Ward Gardner, A., John Wright & Sons, Bristol.)

Geographical	Organizational	Personal
Climate	Nature	Age
Region	Size	Sex
Ethnic	Industrial relations	Occupation
Social insurance	Personnel policy	Job satisfaction
Health services	Sick pay	Personality
Epidemics	Supervisory quality	Life crises
Unemployment	Working conditions	Medical conditions
Social attitudes	Environmental hazards	Alcohol
Pension age	Occupational health service	Family responsibility
	Labour turnover	Journey to work
		Social activities

165

Table 17.2. International sickness absence ratios: per capita rates for 1967, 1968 and 1969 expressed as percentages of mean rates for 1955 and 1956. (After Taylor, P. J. (1972). *Proc. Roy. Soc. Med.* **65**, 577.)

Country	Frequency (spells)			Severity (days)			Estimated average no. of calendar days of absence per person for 1968
	1967	1968	1969	1967	1968	1969	
Great Britain	129	133	138	110*	121*	125*	15
West Germany	109	130	138	115	129	136	15
Sweden	205	225	255	140	151	164	18
The Netherlands	121	126	145	135	152	168	21
Italy	134	146	147	138	195	195	14
Czechoslovakia	95	105	110	79	76	91	16
Yugoslavia	NA	NA	NA	93	93	100	12
Poland	NA	NA	NA	109	98	115	15
U.S.A.	NA	NA	NA	131[†]	137[†]	139[†]	—

* Years ending in June.
[†] No. of persons losing some time in the week surveyed on a weekly sample basis.
NA = not available.

omission from this list is the effects of alcohol abuse because patients often conceal it from doctors and doctors often conceal it from employers.

The longer the spell of sickness absence the greater the relative importance of disease. In short-term sickness absence, lasting a few days only, social factors are a prominent influence in the decision of the worker to stay away from work and declare himself 'sick' and his subsequent decision to return to work. Those who are off for a longer period are usually suffering from a chronic disabling disease (Table 17.4).

About one-third of all sickness absence in males is due to four conditions: hypertensive disease, ischaemic heart disease, chronic bronchitis and arthritis.

Prevention by disease prevention

One way to prevent sickness absence is to prevent the diseases that cause it, e.g. the number of days lost because of pulmonary

Table 17.3. Certified days of male incapacity per 100 at risk aged 20–64 years by diagnostic group for 1954–5 and 1978–9, in Great Britain.

Diagnosis	Days per 100 men at risk	
	1954–5	1978–9
Sprains and strains	9.4	51.4
Nervousness, debility, headache	9.5	59.7
Ill-defined symptoms	36.7	73.8
Psychoneurosis and psychoses	107.6	160.3*
Displacement of intervertebral disc	10.3	32.3
Eczema and dermatitis	12.5	9.1
Cellulitis	10.7	4.7
Arteriosclerosis and degenerative heart disease	64.4	150.7†
Other forms of heart disease	24.7	34.0
Hypertensive disease	26.4	59.0
Varicose veins	7.0	6.8
Neoplasms	9.1	11.6
Acute tonsilitis	10.6	4.7
Pneumonia	11.3	3.1
Bronchitis	144.3	171.1
Stomach and duodenal ulcer	42.7	22.0‡
Gastritis and duodenitis	22.1	15.1
Hernia of abdominal cavity	17.6	22.1
Diarrhoea and enteritis	9.5	23.3
Appendicitis	8.5	3.4
TB of respiratory system	104.8	9.0
Asthma	20.0	11.8
Arthritis	43.9	125.8§
Rheumatism	51.6	30.3**
All causes	1330	1908

* Mental disorders in 1978–9.
† Acute myocardial infarct, chronic and other ischaemic heart disease in 1978–9.
‡ Stomach, duodenal and peptic ulcer in 1978–9.
§ Osteo, allied conditions, other arthritis and spondylitis in 1978–9.
** Rheumatism and lumbago in 1978–9.

tuberculosis in 1978–9 was only 7.3% of the days lost in 1954–5. There is obviously scope for preventing sickness absence by the prevention of stroke, chronic bronchitis and ischaemic heart disease.

Table 17.4. Principal causes of long-term sickness absence in 1972–3. (After Martin, J. & Morgan, M. (1975) *Prolonged Sickness Absence and the Return to Work.* HMSO, London.)

Percentage of people off work for 6 months	Type of disease
31 ●●●●●●●●●●●●●●●●●●●●●●●●●●●●●●●	Heart and circulatory
18 ●●●●●●●●●●●●●●●●●	Bone and joint
17 ●●●●●●●●●●●●●●●●	Respiratory
16 ●●●●●●●●●●●●●●●	Result of accident
12 ●●●●●●●●●●●	Mental
10 ●●●●●●●●●	Digestive

Prevention by effective treatment

One of the objectives of medical intervention is to return the ill person to work as quickly as possible. The provision of effective treatment without undue delay to the worker who is off sick has a part to play in minimizing sickness absence. This applies particularly to the treatment of soft-tissue injuries ('sprains and strains'), arthritis and rheumatism, and backache. For this reason some employers provide physiotherapy at work as part of the occupational-health service; there have also been calls for those who are off sick to be given preferential treatment by the NHS. Waiting lists are not separated into the employed and the unemployed, but the effect of the disease on a person's ability to work does influence the decisions made by a doctor when considering a patient's need for treatment; for example it influences the timing of an admission for a hernia operation.

Prevention by social engineering

A large number of social factors affect the individual's decisions concerning staying off, or returning to work when they feel unwell. However, only some of these can be influenced by employers.
1 Working conditions, e.g. temperature of the working environment.
2 Industrial relations.
3 Personal policy.
4 Sick pay.

5 Supervisory quality.
6 Occupational health service available to staff.
7 Job satisfaction.

Improving the physical conditions

Although it is obviously important to improve adverse physical conditions, e.g. temperatures that are too high or too low, a dusty environment or a noisy workplace, the improvement in sickness absence rate or productivity (for sickness absence rates change in line with other measures of a firm's efficiency) which can be brought about by improving the physical environment is limited (Fig. 17.1).

Furthermore, one fascinating experiment showed that if the adverse physical environment which had been improved was allowed to develop again, the sickness absence rate did not return to its previous levels (Fig. 17.2). The effect of the change itself, of the employers demonstrating concern about the working conditions of their employees, appeared to have been important. This effect—known as the Hawthorne effect because it was demonstrated in a Hawthorne Electric Company factory—shows that social factors in the work place are important as well as social factors at home. Indeed, it has been argued that if social conditions are improved, changes in sickness absence rate or produc-

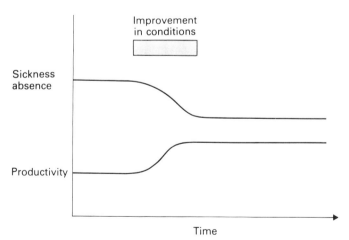

Fig. 17.1. Decline in sickness and absence, and improvement in productivity following improvement of the physical environment.

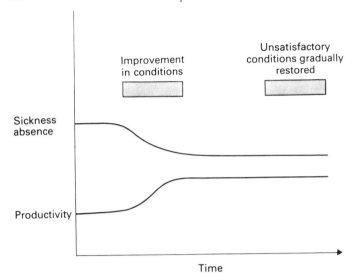

Sickness absence

Productivity

Improvement in conditions

Unsatisfactory conditions gradually restored

Time

Fig. 17.2. Maintenance of reduced sickness absence and enhanced productivity even when improvements in the physical environment are allowed to fade away.

tivity do not level out as they do when the only improvements are changes in the physical conditions.

There are two main ways of improving the social environment at work: increasing worker participation and improving job satisfaction.

Increasing worker participation

Firms or businesses in which the employees play an active part in the management have a lower sickness absence rate than those in which the workers' views are not considered seriously. This does not necessarily mean that the appointment of workers to sit on the Board will reduce sickness absence rates and improve productivity. What is needed is the involvement of the work-force in all decisions affecting their health and well-being, e.g. decisions about the procedures used in dealing with people who are frequently off sick for short periods, in working out the principles of a new shift system, or in the evolution of a policy to help people who are developing problems caused by alcohol abuse.

Improving job satisfaction

Whatever its type, those who are satisfied with their job are off sick less frequently than the person who is dissatisfied. If the satisfied worker does go off sick he is likely to return more quickly than the dissatisfied worker.

Whatever the nature of the job, a worker's satisfaction can be increased by the following measures:

1 as much freedom as possible to organize the job and his working day;

2 recognition and reward for good performance;

3 scope for innovation;

4 opportunities for promotion;

5 opportunities to identify with the end-product.

Prevention of occupational disease and injuries

Occupational diseases and injuries are those caused by the work itself. The common industrial diseases are:

1 occupational dermatitis–over 850 000 working days are lost from skin disease caused by irritation or allergy;

2 pneumoconiosis due to the inhalation of particles—more than 40 000 people receive social security benefits because they have pneumoconiosis; most of them are coal miners affected by silicosis;

3 accidents—there are nearly half a million accidents at work every year, of which about 1 000 are fatal.

Certain occupational diseases are called 'prescribed diseases' because they are prescribed under the National Insurance (Industrial Injuries) Act of 1946. If a disease is prescribed the person is automatically entitled to receive financial help from the state. He neither has to prove that the employer was negligible nor that he could not have contracted the disease at home. Examples of prescribed diseases are:

1 mesothelioma in asbestos workers;

2 bladder cancer in workers who have been working with B naphthylamine;

3 tuberculosis in those who have been caring for an infected person, or who have been handling tuberculous material in a laboratory.

The Health and Safety at Work Act 1974

The prevention of industrial disease has a long legislative history. A large number of Acts of Parliament were passed in both the nineteenth and the twentieth centuries. All these Acts, some covering many workers, some only protecting a small number, were gathered together under a consolidating Act in 1974–the Health and Safety at Work Act. This Act also provided legal protection for about eight million workers who had previously had no legal cover, and it spelled out the general principles on which health and safety at work were to be promoted. It states that, 'it shall be the duty of every employer to ensure, so far as is reasonably practicable, the health, safety and welfare at work of all his employees'. It also states that it shall be the 'duty of every employee while at work to take reasonable care of himself and of other people who may be affected by his acts or omissions'. Implementation of the Act is carried out by the Health and Safety Executive, part of which is the Employment Medical Advisory Service consisting of occupational health doctors and nurses. The Executive is supervised by the Health and Safety Commission appointed by the Secretary of State for Employment.

The employer has to nominate safety officers to be responsible for the health and safety of employees. These are usually departmental heads, but many larger firms also have a full-time specialist safety officer. The trades unions nominate safety representatives to sit with the safety officers on the safety committee.

Although this appears a neat and simple system, the interpretation of the Act and its implementation have proved difficult and it is not surprising that there has been no significant decline in the numbers of industrial diseases or accidents since 1974. Nevertheless, the Act does represent an advance in the prevention of occupational diseases and injuries.

Occupational health services

The provision of occupational health services varies widely: some employers employ full-time medical and nursing staff, others have none at all, the main deciding factor being the size of the firm. Small firms employing less than 250 people usually do not have either a medical service or an occupational health nurse, whereas those which employ more than 1000 people often employ both doctors and nurses.

Occupational medicine has a very wide scope because the range of different types of job is so vast, but the functions of doctors and nurses working in occupational health departments can be grouped under prevention, helping workers adjust to their jobs and treatment.

Prevention

There are two aspects of preventive work. The main preventive function is to try to detect and prevent occupational disease, i.e. disease which is caused by the work the employee is required to do or by risks to which he is exposed in the course of his work. It is, however, difficult for an individual doctor or nurse to identify new health hazards for a number of reasons.

1 In most firms the number of employed is too small for new epidemics to be observed, particularly if the disease is uncommon and only affects a small proportion of workers.

2 Many people change jobs frequently so that an individual's job when he develops a disease may be different from the work which caused it.

3 The delay between exposure to a risk and the development of disease can be so long that the person may have retired before disease develops.

For these reasons much of the basic epidemiological research is carried out in academic departments, and the task of the occupational health staff becomes the implementation of preventive measures, rather than the detection of new risks and hazards, although accident patterns and epidemics of dermatitis can be identified in a factory.

Occupational health staff do this work in cooperation with the full-time safety officer and with the training department of the firm, for the education of staff is of vital importance in the prevention of occupational diseases.

In addition to these specific preventive measures some occupational health departments also offer general preventive services, e.g. cervical cytology or multiphasic screening of senior staff, but these can only be offered by departments which are confident that they have covered all the aspects of prevention relating to hazards arising directly from the work itself.

Adjustment to work
There are three ways in which occupational health staff can help people adjust to the work they wish to do or have to do.
1 Pre-employment screening, with the intention of dissuading applicants from jobs for which they are unsuited, e.g. dissuading people who have a history of backache from jobs that involve lifting.
2 Helping employees who have become disabled to find alternative work they can do and, in discussion with the Disablement Resettlement Officer (DRO), helping disabled people find jobs that they can do in spite of their disability.
3 Counselling people who have been off sick for a large number of short periods, or for a single long period of time.

These aspects of occupational medicine pose some extremely difficult problems for doctors and nurses because the occupational health service has to remain completely independent of both management and the trades unions and has to be seen as such by both sides.

Treatment
Many occupational services provide treatment of both emergencies and chronic conditions, e.g. soft-tissue injuries, which require physiotherapy. Treatment services are important, not only because they can help employees to return to work but also because they increase the confidence of staff in the occupational health service. They thus provide a better basis for its preventive efforts and establish trust, which helps the doctors and nurses when they are giving advice about an individual's fitness to work. Occupational health doctors and nurses obviously need expertise but they also need the trust and confidence of management and trades unions.

CHAPTER 18
CANCER

Generalizations about cancer are fraught with difficulties because there are so many different types of neoplasm, but there are common themes in the research and prevention of cancers, an important one being their preventability. Epidemiological studies suggest that almost all cancers have exterior causes and that very few have internal causes, such as genetic factors or the effects of the ageing process. At present only about one-third of cancers have had their causes identified (Table 18.1), but estimates have been made of the proportion of cancer deaths that will ultimately be found to be attributable to external factors (Table 18.2) and it is estimated that virtually all will have external causes and will therefore be preventable.

It is thus possible to develop a cancer-prevention strategy, even though the causes of all the cancers are not known. The basis of a cancer-prevention strategy based on the causal factors is outlined in Table 18.3.

The advances in cancer epidemiology have been considerable but the gaps remain large and more research is necessary. This is

Table 18.1. Reliably established (as of 1981), practicable* ways of avoiding the onset of life-threatening cancer with the percentage of all U.S. cancer deaths known to be thus avoidable

Avoidance of tobaco smoke	30
Avoidance of alcoholic drinks or mouthwashes	3
Avoidance of obesity	2
Regular cervical screening and genital hygiene	1
Avoidance of inessential medical use of hormones or radiology	< 1
Avoidance of unusual exposure to sunlight	< 1
Avoidance of current levels of exposure to currently known effects of carcinogens (for which there is good epidemiological evidence of human hazard) in:	
the occupational context;	< 1
food, water or urban air	< 1

* Excluding ways such as prophylactic prostatectomy, mastectomy, hysterectomy, oophorectomy, artifical menopause or pregnancy.

175

Table 18.2. Estimate of the proportions of all U.S. cancer deaths that will be found to be attributable to various factors [†]

Factor	Best estimate (%)	Range of acceptable estimate (%)
Tobacco	30	25–40
Alcohol	3	2–4
Diet	35	10–70
Food additives	<1	−5*–2
Sexual behaviour	1	1
Yet-to-be-discovered hormonal analogues of reproductive factors	−6	−112–0
Occupation	4	2–8
Pollution	2	1–5
Industrial products	<1	<1–2
Medicines and medical procedures	1	0.5–3
Geophysical factors (mostly natural background radiation and sunlight)	3	2–4
Infective processes	10?	1–?
Unknown	?[†]	?
Total	200 or more[†]	

* The net effects of food additives may be protective, e.g. against stomach cancer.
[†] Since one cancer may have two or more causes, the grand total in such a table will probably, when more knowledge is available, greatly exceed 200%. (It is merely a coincidence that the suggested figures in the present table happen to add up to nearly 100%.) Peto, R. (1981) The Times Health Supplement, 6 Nov, pp. 12–14.

funded both by Government and by the large cancer charities, notably the Imperial Cancer Research Fund and the Cancer Research Campaign. International effort is coordinated by WHO and the Union International Contre le Cancer (UICC).

Prevention of specific cancers

In addition to a preventive strategy orientated towards risk factors it is also necessary to think of cancer prevention in terms of a disease, identifying the different cancers and working out a preventive strategy for each one. The actions of such a strategy are summarized in Table 18.4 using the three stages described in Chapter 4.

There is, in addition, a need for education of the public about

Table 18.3. Cancer prevention strategy

Causal factor	Preventive strategy	Responsible bodies in U.K. other than Department of Health
Tobacco	Measures designed to stop young people starting to smoke and to help smokers to stop	Health Education Council Scottish Health Education Group Action on Smoking and Health
Alcohol	Measures designed to reduce alcohol abuse	Health Education Council Scottish Health Education Group
Diet	Need for more epidemiological research	Cancer charities funding research
Food additives	Regulations to test and control food additives Food labelling to allow consumer choice	Department of Prices and Consumer Protection
Sexual behaviour	Education about sexual hygiene Promotion of the use of 'barrier' methods of contraception	Staff working in family-planning services
Occupational factors and the presence of carcinogens in industrial products	Continued research on occupational mortality rates to detect risk factors Implementation of principles laid down in Health and Safety at Work Act	Health and Safety Executive
Pollution	Increased environmental monitoring to detect new pollutants Pollution control	Department of the Environment Environmental Health Committees of local authorities
Medicines	Maintenance of system of notification of drug effects and rigorous testing of new drugs	Committee on Safety of Medicines
Geophysical factors	Research into geographical variations in cancer incidence Advice on hazards of sun-bathing	Cancer charities funding research
Infective processes	Need for increased research	Cancer charities funding research

Table 18.4. Three stage cancer prevention

Stage	Action
Primary prevention	Education of those at risk about steps they can take Control of risk factors by modification of the social and physical environment
Secondary prevention	Screening—the detection of the cancer at a pre-symptomatic stage
Tertiary prevention	Public education to encourage early presentation Professional education to promote early diagnosis and effective treatment

cancer in general because the prevailing belief of many people is still that cancer is an incurable disease with a hopeless prognosis. Many professionals are also still too pessimistic. It is essential to promote a more positive, hopeful attitude towards cancer in

Table 18.5. Neoplasms: numbers of deaths and cumulative percentage of deaths from various sites in the population of England and Wales in 1978

Site	No. deaths	Cumulative %
Males		
Lung	26 925	39.2
Stomach	6 698	48.9
Prostate	4 730	55.8
Large intestine	4 324	62.1
Rectum	3 202	66.8
Pancreas	3 008	71.2
Bladder	2 951	75.5
Oesophagus	2 085	78.5
Leukaemia	1 832	81.2
Brain tumours	1 761	83.7
Females		
Breast	11 915	20.1
Lung	7 606	32.9
Large intestine	6 057	43.1
Stomach	4 799	51.2
Ovaries and fallopian tubes	3 784	57.6
Rectum	2 847	62.4
Pancreas	2 692	66.9
Uterus, cervix	2 153	68.9
Oesophagus	1 623	73.3
Uterus, others	1 567	75.9

Source: Alderson, M. (1982) *The Prevention of Cancer*, p. 5. Arnold, London.

which the specific strategies can be developed. Cancer education, such as that promoted by the UICC (Union Internationale Contre le Cancer), has an important part to play in prevention.

Priorities in cancer prevention

Although there are many different types of cancer, more than four-fifths of cancer deaths in men and more than three-quarters of those in women are caused by no more than ten types of cancers (Table 18.5). Six are common to both lists, so there are fourteen types of cancer responsible for about four-fifths of all cancer deaths, i.e. about 100 000 deaths per annum in England and Wales (Table 18.6).

Research

Of these fourteen there are seven in which there is insufficient knowledge to allow any programme of primary or secondary prevention to be planned. The priority for these cancers is therefore more epidemiological research (Table 18.7).

Smoking

Cancer of the lung, pancreas and oesophagus are known to be

Table 18.6. The fourteen types of cancer responsible for four-fifths of all cancer deaths

Site of cancer	Priorities for prevention	No. dying annually in England and Wales
Stomach Prostate Brain Ovary Breast Rectum Large intestine	Insufficient evidence for effective primary or secondary prevention: priority for more epidemiological research	50 000
Lung Pancreas Oesophagus	Priority prevention of cigarette smoking Alcohol abuse also important	43 000
Cervix Bladder Leukaemia Body of uterus	Evidence to allow primary and secondary preventive measures: priority development of effective services	8 000

Table 18.7. Cancers for which there is insufficient evidence to mount primary or secondary prevention programmes

Site of cancer	Comments
Stomach	Incidence falling in Western countries for no known reason There has been a screening programme for 20 years in Japan where the incidence is much higher, using double-contrast barium meal but screening has not been adequately evaluated
Prostate	There has been a two-fold increase in male mortality this century in England but no cause has yet been identified
Brain	There has been a steady increase in mortality this century, some of this probably being due to more accurate diagnosis
Ovary	Increase in mortality this century There is evidence that there is an increased risk in women first having intercourse, being pregnant at the age of 20, having few children or having an early menopause, i.e. evidence it is related to hormonal changes
Breast	There is experimental evidence that screening saves lives but there is not yet sufficient evidence to introduce a screening service
Rectum and large intestine	Dietary factors are obviously suspected but none have yet been identified Screening for large bowel cancer by testing for blood in the faeces is currently being examined

Source: Chamberlain, J. (1982) In *The Prevention of Cancer* (ed. M. Alderson), pp. 259–284. Arnold, London.

caused by cigarette smoking. There are, therefore, no specific strategies for the prevention of these cancers other than the prevention of smoking and the prevention of alcohol abuse for oesophageal cancer.

Development of specific services

Thus, there remain only four cancers for which there are specific preventive strategies in the U.K., i.e. those affecting the bladder, blood, uterus and cervix. Causes and preventive measures for these are given in Table 18.8.

There is therefore considerable scope for prevention, particularly through the prevention of cigarette smoking.

Table 18.8. Cancers which can be prevented by specific services

	Bladder cancer	Leukaemia	Cancer of body of uterus	Cancer of cervix
Principal causal factors	Smoking Certain chemicals used in rubber and dye industries	Ionizing radiation	High doses of oestrogen	Unknown, possibly viral
Primary prevention	Measures to prevent smoking Substitution of carcinogenic chemicals by harmless ones Industrial safety measures	Education of doctors to minimize the numbers of X-rays taken, especially in pregnancy	Caution in prescribing oestrogen as hormone-replacement therapy	Education about the need for genital hygiene and the protective benefits of barrier contraceptives
Secondary prevention	Cytological examination of urine specimens of workers at regular intervals	Film badges for those working with radiation Medical examination of designated radiation workers	Close medical supervision of women receiving hormone-replacement therapy	Cervical smear test
Responsible authority	Department of Health and Social Security	National Radiological Protection Board	No authority is responsible. The responsibility is the medical profession's	District Health Authorities
Obstacles to prevention	Low coverage of screening programme	Increasing use of radioactive materials	Unrestrained use of oestrogens in some countries	Poorly organized service in U.K.

CHAPTER 19
HEART ATTACKS AND STROKES

Introduction

The main cause of death in developed countries is arterial disease, particularly coronary heart disease and cerebrovascular disease. Together these two conditions account for roughly half of all deaths (Fig. 19.1), and coronary heart disease alone accounts for almost half of all deaths in middle-aged men. It has been suggested that, by the application of existing knowledge, about half of all strokes and a quarter of all deaths from coronary heart disease in people under 70 could probably be prevented.

The 'epidemic' of coronary heart disease seems to have begun in the 1930s and within 20 years to have become by far the most common cause of premature death. Mortality continued to rise and between 1950 and 1970 the death rate from coronary heart disease amongst men in Britain almost doubled. Since then there

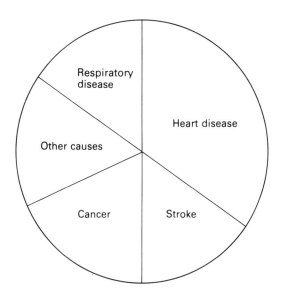

Fig. 19.1. Causes of death in the U.K.

has been a levelling off and some suggestion recently of a slight fall. In the U.S.A. and Australia, death rates from coronary heart disease fell by 25% in the decade 1968–77 (Fig. 19.2).

There has also been a change in the social class distribution of coronary heart disease, changes which are almost certainly due to shifts in behaviour. Until the 1950s deaths from coronary heart disease occurred more frequently in upper- and middle-class men than in working-class men. However, by 1970 this had changed considerably, and death rates from coronary heart

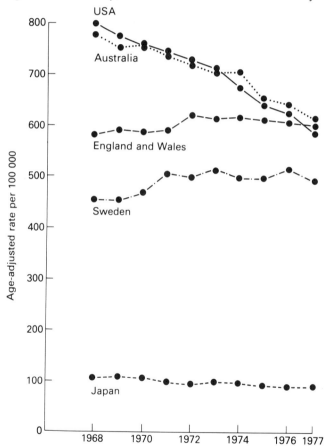

Fig. 19.2. Ischaemic heart disease mortality in males aged 35–74 years in the U.S.A., Australia, England and Wales, Sweden and Japan. (After Marmot *et al.* (1981) *Health Trends*, Vol. 13. HMSO, London.)

disease were 12% below average in professionals and 11% above average in unskilled labourers. The change in the social-class pattern is even more evident in the younger age group, with deaths from coronary heart disease in males aged 35–44 years being 75% below the average in professionals and 55% above the average amongst unskilled labourers. These social-class differences are probably the main explanation for the large differences in coronary heart disease mortality in different parts of Britain (Fig. 19.3).

There appears to have been no 'epidemic' of cerebrovascular disease comparable to that of coronary heart disease, but mortal-

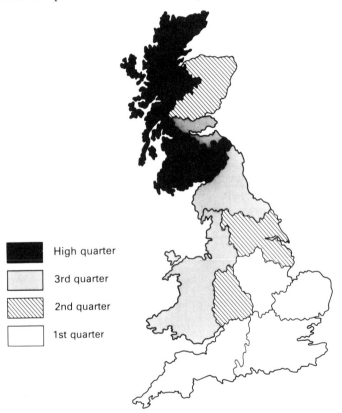

High quarter

3rd quarter

2nd quarter

1st quarter

Fig. 19.3. Death rates for ischaemic heart disease in males aged 45–54 years in the standard regions of England, Wales and Scotland, divided by quartiles. (After Fulton *et al.* (1978) *Br. Heart J.* 40, 566.)

ity from stroke is declining and there has again been a change in the social-class pattern. In the 1950s there was no significant social-class difference in deaths from cerebrovascular disease. Since then, however, a steep gradient has opened up so that by 1970 mortality from cerebrovascular disease in professional men was 30% below average and that in unskilled labourers more than 50% above average.

Coronary heart disease

Risk factors
Many epidemiological and other studies have clearly established important risk factors for coronary heart disease. The major ones are:
1 cigarette smoking;
2 raised blood pressure;
3 elevated blood lipids.
Others include:
1 diabetes;
2 physical inactivity;
3 Type A personality;
4 obesity (but whether this is an important independent risk factor is debatable).

Another important risk factor is that of a family history of coronary heart disease, especially at an early age. Although there is nothing reversible about this, its importance lies in finding those in whom the identification and management of other risk factors is particularly worthwhile.

The major risk factors are frequently associated one with another, so that more than half the coronary heart disease and sudden heart deaths occur in the 20% or so of individuals with two or more of them. Beyond reasonable doubt these risk factors are causal and their control can influence coronary heart disease mortality.

Cigarette smoking is the risk factor which demonstrates the best evidence of reversibility. In the British Doctors' Study mortality from coronary heart disease was halved within 5 years in cigarette smokers who stopped, and half this benefit occurred in the first year. Those who have already suffered myocardial infarction benefit more from stopping smoking than from any other single measure, reducing the risk of death from subsequent infarction by 50% compared with those who continue to smoke.

The mortality rate from coronary heart disease for smokers is about twice that of non-smokers, but this apparently modest effect of smoking conceals two important considerations. One is the importance of coronary heart disease from which about 150 000 people die each year in Britain, a quarter of them under the age of 65 years. The other is the disproportionately greater risk in the younger age group: under the age of 45 years the smoking of twenty-five or more cigarettes daily is associated with a fifteen times greater risk than non-smokers of dying from coronary heart disease.

Coronary heart disease in women is less common than men, but mortality from this cause in women is increasing. Smoking greatly increases the risk of coronary heart disease associated with taking the combined oral contraceptive pill and, although this risk is not significant in young women, older women on the pill who smoke thirty-five or more cigarettes daily have a twenty-fold greater risk of myocardial infarction than non-smokers.

The mechanisms whereby smoking causes coronary heart disease are unclear, but increased coronary atheroma has been demonstrated in smokers, as has increased platelet stickiness, increased concentration of fibrinogen and other coagulation factors, and an increased tendency to arrhythmias in response to catecholamines. (Many sudden heart deaths, especially in the younger age group, are probably due to arrhythmias, post-mortems on such patients demonstrating severe atheroma but no actual arterial occlusion.)

Although low-tar cigarettes have been shown to be less damaging to the lungs than high-tar ones (so that their introduction has contributed to the decline in lung cancer in men), neither this change nor the switch from plain to filter cigarettes appear to have reduced the risk of coronary heart disease in smokers. There is even some suggestion that filter cigarettes may be worse in this respect than plain ones. (It is known that filter cigarettes yield more carbon monoxide.)

There is no doubt therefore about the importance of smoking as a cause of coronary heart disease, nor about the benefits of stopping. There is much less certainty about how to avoid smoking or achieve smoking cessation (see Chapter 12).

Raised blood pressure is also a clearly established risk factor for coronary heart disease. However, the evidence of benefit from the treatment of hypertension in the prevention of coronary heart disease is less clear than is the case with smoking. This may be because of failure to treat high blood pressure at an early enough stage. There is some evidence of falls in coronary heart disease mortality following treatment of mild to moderate hypertension and, because this is such a common risk factor (affecting up to 20% of the middle-aged population), the potential preventive yield from control of this factor could be very substantial. Whether this might be achieved by medication, behavioural approaches or reduction of dietary sodium (see Chapter 11), remains debatable.

Elevated blood lipids is the third major risk factor for coronary heart disease. Many epidemiological studies have demonstrated a clear relationship between diet and coronary heart disease risk, probably through an effect on both atherosclerosis and thrombosis. Several aspects of the 'Western diet' (see Chapter 11) are thought to be contributory. However, as with raised blood pressure, the evidence of benefit from intervention is not conclusive. Again this is probably because if changes are to be effective they need to be implemented early in life.

In population studies there are strong associations between saturated fat intake (and plasma cholesterol levels) and coronary heart disease death rates. In an early study of the relation between diet and deaths from ischaemic heart disease in seven countries, Keys* showed that there were strong positive correlations with the amount of saturated fat and dietary sugar eaten and that blood cholesterol concentrations were strongly related to the proportion of calorie intake contributed by saturated fat. Other studies showed that migrating populations, e.g. Japanese moving to California, in adapting a higher fat intake also acquired a higher incidence of ischaemic heart disease. More recently an intervention study, the Oslo Heart Study, a controlled trial in which dietary and smoking advice was studied prospectively,

*Keys, A. (1980) *Seven Countries: A Multivariate Analysis of Death and Coronary Heart Disease*. Harvard University Press, Cambridge.

has shown a reduction in coronary heart deaths in men who reduced their fat intake.

There is little evidence that specific cholesterol-lowering diets are any more effective than diets aimed simply at reducing body weight to within 10% of the optimal. This requires the adoption of a prudent or natural diet with calorie intake restricted to that necessary to maintain optimal weight, fats limited to 30% of total energy intake and a dietary fibre intake of 30 g a day (see Chapter 11).

Although these three factors—cigarette smoking, high blood pressure and hyperlipidaemia—are the outstanding risk factors for coronary heart disease, others are probably contributory.

Exercise may have a protective effect, apart from any benefit it may have in the control of obesity (and hence hyperlipidaemia) or on blood pressure. Retrospective studies show lower coronary risk for those taking regular, vigorous exercise.

Personality is also associated with coronary risk. Aggressive, competitive individuals (so called Type A personalities) appear to be at greater risk than the more phlegmatic (so called Type B) individuals. Acute stress and adverse life events may also be associated with increased risk.

Although less important in themselves, the last three factors assume enhanced significance in those who have major risk factors for coronary heart disease.

Prevention

There is now some evidence that screening for major coronary risk factors and their correction on a population basis may be beneficial in reducing the incidence of and mortality from coronary heart disease. Therefore, although no controlled trials have demonstrated the benefits of such screening and intervention in general practice, there is now a strong case for such activity on a case-finding basis. Those with a family history of cardiovascular disease, particularly coronary heart disease at an early age in the parents or siblings, should be subject to special scrutiny. Cigarette smoking, high blood pressure and obesity should be ascertained and where possible remedied.

Smoking is a major target. Many have stopped smoking and

others can be helped to do so (see Chapter 12). Smoking needs to be treated as a clinical problem in its own right with the elicitation of a history and management of the condition being treated as the serious clinical problem it is. At the present time, only a small proportion of clinical records in general practice have any indication of smoking status.

Raised blood pressure needs also to be more effectively detected and managed. At the present time, as the 'Rule of Halves' (Fig. 19.4) acknowledges, only half of those with hypertension are known, half of those identified are on treatment and only half of those effectively controlled. Less than half the general practice records of middle-aged men provide evidence of blood pressure having been recorded within the last 10 years. There is therefore scope for considerable improvement here, and a good case now for treatment of an individual below the age of 65 years who has a blood pressure of 180/100 or above, as the mean of three readings.

Obesity is a visible target and a reliable indicator of raised blood lipids. Like smoking, the weighing of patients needs to be acknowledged as a respectable clinical activity, as does the offer

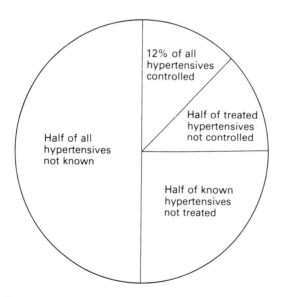

Fig. 19.4. The 'Rule of Halves' for hypertension.

of advice and support to those who need to lose weight (see Chapter 11). Using the measurement of blood pressure as a cue to enquire about smoking and to record weight may not only facilitate the performance of these two latter activities by the doctor, but encourage the patient to see them as important to health.

Diabetes is a condition which substantially increases the risk of coronary heart disease. Diabetics, like those with a strong family history of coronary heart disease, require special supervision with attention to coronary risk factors. Present evidence suggests there is much scope for improving such monitoring of diabetics in general practice.

Implementation of recommendations

As usual, there is a gap between knowledge and its application. This is nowhere more true than in the prevention of Western society's major killer. Major changes are required in the behaviour of both doctors and their patients. However, as described in the introduction to this chapter, there have been substantial reductions in coronary heart disease deaths in some countries. Although it is difficult to define the precise causation, it seems clear that reduced smoking, dietary changes, improved detection and management of high blood pressure and more exercise have contributed to this. In Britain, similar changes are now taking place.

General practice has a major role to play in achieving the reduction in coronary heart disease which current knowledge makes possible. But the anticipatory care necessary is a new concept to doctors who have become accustomed to responding only to patients' symptoms and complaints.

Opportunities for prevention arise during normal care and there are such opportunities in almost every consultation. The potential of the general practice consultation for health education and preventive activities has been well described: each consultation offers the opportunity not only for dealing with the problem presented, but also for wide health care, i.e.:
1 the modification of help-seeking behaviour;
2 the management of continuing problems;
3 opportunistic health promotion.

Doctors seem generally to be diffident about discussing health promotion and prevention with their patients, but should remind themselves that the Latin origin of the word doctor is teacher. It has been shown that 'of all the many and varied sources of health information available to the adult population, it is the general practitioner who is most trusted and whose advice has most impact'* and evidence of the effectiveness of advice from the GP is available at least in relation to smoking (see Chapter 12).

Effective prevention will therefore depend on the willingness of doctors to advise on such things as smoking, diet, alcohol intake, exercise and on the willingness of patients to comply with and implement such advice. The more clinical activity of detecting raised blood pressure may provide the cue to offer such advice.

Cerebrovascular disease

Risk factors

High blood pressure is the outstanding risk factor for strokes. Epidemiological studies show that below the age of 70, risk increases with systolic and diastolic pressures and that the former is a better predictor than the latter. What is more, there is good evidence that reduction of blood pressure substantially reduces the risk of stroke and although debate continues about the 'cut-off point' above which treatment is of proven benefit, there is a consensus that treatment of sustained blood pressure of 180/100 or above in the age range 35–70 years is beneficial. However the major initial task is the detection of those with high blood pressure. This needs to be supplemented by systematic management and follow-up of those hypertensives detected.

The most obvious way of ascertaining hypertension is by a case-finding approach in general practice. Up to two-thirds of adults consult a GP at least once a year and over 90% at least once every 5 years. Given that measurement of blood pressure adds approximately 1 minute only to the consultation, the feasibility of this would seem reasonable. But it is important that blood

*McCron, R. & Budd, J. *Communication and health education,* Chapter 8. Prepared for the Health Education Council, October 1979 (unpublished). University of Leicester Centre for Mass Communication Research.

pressure so measured should be recorded in the medical records in such a way that the information is easily accessible; not only so that comparison over time may be made, but also to avoid unnecessary repetition. The aim should be to achieve at least one reading of blood pressure every 5 years in patients aged 35 (or better still 20) to 64 years. Between 5% and 10% of the adult population in this age group will be identified as hypertensive (blood pressure at or above 180/100)—between 50 and 100 patients in the average practice list of a little over 2000. About twice this number will be found to have 'borderline hypertension' (with blood pressures at or above 160/90, but below 180/100). These should have their blood pressures checked yearly. The remainder with blood pressure below 160/90 will need to have blood pressure checks only once every 5 years.

The blood pressure should be recorded in the notes in a place regularly used for that purpose. Some doctors use a 'basic data' sheet which also facilitates recording of other information, such as smoking status and weight, and there is much to be said for this. The notes also need to be 'tagged' in a way which indicates when the next blood-pressure recording is due. The simplest way

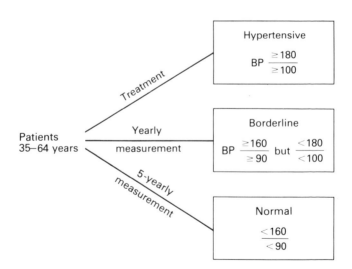

Fig. 19.5. The 'Three box' system for monitoring hypertensive patients on treatment.

to do this is to use a sticker on which is written the date (year and possibly month) when this should be repeated. The sticker can then be superimposed as required.

While this will be a sufficient reminder for those requiring 5-yearly measurement, there is great advantage in establishing a box file system for those hypertensives on treatment (Fig. 19.5). Using this, it is then possible to ensure that regular supervision takes place.

A similar box file system should also be established for the 'borderline hypertensives'. This will not only facilitate the achievement of annual blood-pressure checks, but also make it possible to identify easily this group of patients should evidence become available that they might benefit from treatment.

Much of the work involved in case-finding and follow-up can be done by a practice nurse and a protocol suitable for use in this context is illustrated in Fig. 19.6.

Other risk factors for stroke are smoking and raised blood lipids but, relative to blood pressure, they seem to be less important than they are in relation to coronary heart disease. Smoking doubles the risk at least in men, and is more important in the younger age group.

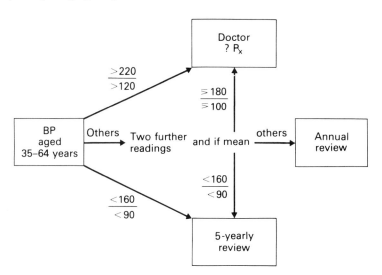

Fig. 19.6. Nurse blood pressure protocol.

Diabetics are at greatly increased risk of cardiovascular disease, stroke included.

Prevention

The claim that half the strokes currently occurring can be prevented by the application of existing knowledge, presents a major challenge. Although achievement of such an objective may seem remote, pursuit of the relatively simple task of detecting those in the community at risk because of undisputed hypertension should be possible. Modern treatments have made the management of raised blood pressure simpler for doctors and more tolerable for patients. However, the task of ensuring proper treatment and follow-up should not be underestimated, nor should the difficulties of encouraging compliance in individuals who, although at risk of major disease, are usually asymptomatic.

CHAPTER 20
PREVENTION OF PHYSICAL DISABILITY AND HANDICAP

The World Health Organization has agreed on definitions for the terms 'impairment', 'disability' and 'handicap'.

TERM	MEANING	EXAMPLE
Disease	Pathological process	Rheumatoid arthritis
↓	↓	↓
Impairment	Specific physical damage caused by disease	Damage to joints
↓	↓	↓
Disability	Limitations caused by impairment: limitations of functions such as gripping and limitations of activities such as washing oneself	Difficulty with walking Inability to lift heavy objects
↓	↓	↓
Handicap	Loss of satisfactory social role caused by disability	Educational difficulties Unemployment Poverty Inability to enjoy an ordinary social life Dependence on other people for the performance of tasks that most people can perform for themselves

Useful though this WHO classification is, it is important to remember that people can be handicapped without being dis-

Table 20.1. Prevention of impairment, disability and handicap

Means of prevention	Responsible authorities
Prevention of impairment	
Prevention of diseases which cause impairment	All authorities responsible for prevention
Effective treatment of diseases which cause impairment and which cannot be prevented	Health services
Prevention of disability in those whose impairment cannot be prevented	
Prevention of the loss of fitness and loss of confidence that often follows immobility and inactivity	Health services helped by voluntary organizations and social-services departments which run day-centres
This requires education of the person with an impairment to do as much as he can for himself and, even more important the education of his family and friends not to do too much for him	Local authorities providing sports facilities for people with disabilities
Both the person with the impairment and his relatives often need help to cope with the emotional effects of disease and impairment	
Prevention of handicap in those whose disability cannot be prevented	
Provision of special services for people with disability	Social services
Accurate assessment of disabled people so that the appropriate range of services for each individual are provided	Housing
	Voluntary services
	Social Security
Education of professionals to ensure that all are aware of the range of services available	Departments of Employment
	Services for disabled people

Responsible professionals	Contribution of doctor or nurse
Health education Medicine Nursing Physiotherapy Road-safety training officers All other professions involved in prevention	Patient education and public education Preventive measures, such as diagnosis and treatment of high blood pressure Accurate diagnosis and appropriate treatment of disease
Medicine Physiotherapy Nursing Medical social workers (play an important part in helping people to accept and cope with disabilities)	Awareness of harmful effects of immobility and inactivity Education of affected person and relatives Sensitivity to emotional consequences of disease and their effects on disability Awareness of skills of other professionals and willingness to involve them
Occupational therapy District-nursing Social-work	Knowledge of range of social services available Willingness to make contact with appropriate services if disabled person is unable to do so

abled, notably as a result of skin disease or any other condition that causes facial disfigurement, because the impairment of the skin may cause severe social problems and make it difficult for the affected person to find work.

The preventive strategy

The prevention of handicap has three steps.
1 Prevention of impairment.
2 Prevention of disability in those people whose impairment cannot be prevented.
3 Prevention of handicap in those people whose disability cannot be prevented.
These three steps are set out in Table 20.1.

Prevention of impairment in childhood

There are three main ways of preventing physical impairment and mental handicap in childhood.

Prevention of the damage caused by low birth weight can be achieved by more sensitive, more effective antenatal care and by the provision of skilled services for those babies that are born with a low weight.

Prevention of genetic, chromosomal and congenital conditions that cause physical impairment or mental handicap, e.g. Down's Syndrome by:
1 genetic counselling services;
2 rubella immunization of all 14-year-old girls;
3 provision of the alpha-pheto protein test for all pregnant women to detect those likely to be carrying a fetus with spina bifida;
4 provision of amniocentesis service for women suspected of carrying a fetus with spina bifida or Down's syndrome. Unfortunately, the principal means of prevention is abortion, which raises ethical problems.

Prevention of childhood accidents by environmental engineering, backed if necessary by legislation and education.

Prevention of impairment in adult life

The main physical causes of severe impairment in adult life are indicated in Fig. 20.1. Of these, the following diseases cannot be prevented: osteoarthritis; rheumatoid arthritis; Parkinson's disease; multiple sclerosis. The prevention of impairment in these conditions therefore depends on:

1 accurate diagnosis;

2 effective treatment;

3 surveillance and support of people on long-term therapy to ensure compliance and prevent drug side-effects and loss of morale;

4 provision of physiotherapy and encouragement of exercise to minimize loss of fitness.

However, several major causes of impairment can be prevented, e.g. stroke, coronary heart disease, chronic obstructive airways disease, and trauma from accidents causing brain damage, amputation and paraplegia.

Prevention of disability

Immobility and inactivity aggravate the impairment caused by disease (Fig.20.2). To prevent disability it is therefore necessary to minimize inactivity and immobility in the following ways.

1 Effective control of symptoms.

2 Provision of physiotherapy so that the person learns what he can do to minimize the effects of immobility and inactivity.

3 Counselling of the affected person to help him come to terms with the fact that he has a chronic disease.

4 Encouragement of the disabled person to take as much exercise and to participate as fully as possible in life.

5 Education of relatives and friends so that they encourage the person with the disability to keep active and so that they do not take over tasks and responsibilities from him.

These approaches can interrupt the vicious circle of disability.

Prevention of handicap

In all the developed countries services have been developed to prevent handicap. The most important are listed in Table 20.2.

The general principle is to try to avoid the segregation of people with disabilities in special schools, workshops or blocks of flats. This is important, not only because it avoids setting people with disabilities apart from society but also because it helps people who are not significantly disabled—for we are all impaired and disabled to some degree—to learn that those who are obviously impaired, by being paraplegic or by having a disfiguring skin disease, are no different from them.

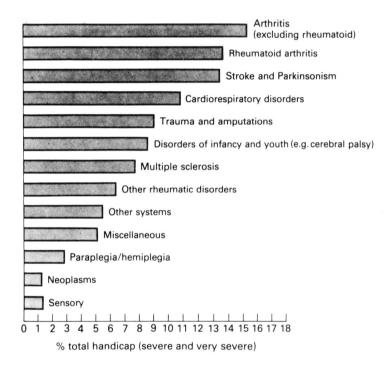

Fig. 20.1. Main physical causes of severe and very severe handicap in adults aged 16–65 years. (After Office of Health Economics (1981) Briefing No. 15. *OHE, London.*)

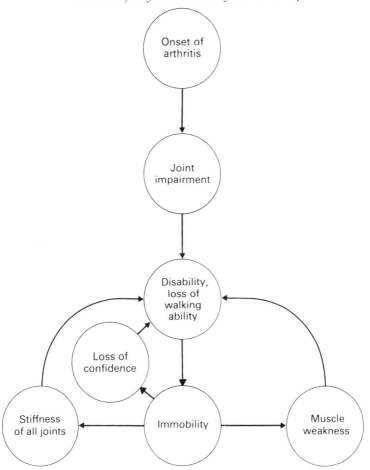

Fig. 20.2. The vicious circle of disability.

Table 20.2. Services for the prevention of handicap

Aims and objectives of service	Responsible authority	Key professionals
Special education		
To prevent educational disadvantages by providing education which takes into account the person's impairment	Health Authority, responsible for assessment Education Authority	Doctors and physiotherapists in child-health services Teachers
Employment		
To help people with disabilities train for and find work	Department of Employment	Disablement Resettlement Officer (DRO)
Housing		
To prevent the handicaps caused by bad house design by: building new dwellings specifically for wheelchair users; designing all dwellings with people who have disabilities in mind; adapting existing dwellings.	Housing Authority Housing Associations (funded directly by Central Government) Social Services Department, which helps with housing adaptations	Architects Housing managers Occupational therapists
Income support		
To prevent poverty	Department of Health and Social Security Local authorities give help with rent and rates	Social workers Advisers in Citizens Advice Bureaux Social security officers
Environmental		
To prevent unnecessary obstacles being placed in the way of people with disabilities who are trying to get work, visit friends or travel to enjoy themselves	Highways Authority Planning departments of local authority Designers of shops, theatres, restaurants and places of entertainment Transport Authority	Designers of buses, trains and planes Highway engineers Architects

CHAPTER 21
PREVENTION OF DENTAL DISEASE

Dental disease is the commonest chronic disease in the U.K. It has three main forms:
1 dental caries—the decay of teeth;
2 periodontal disease—gum disease;
3 the problems of people with no natural teeth.
Both dental caries and peridontal disease are caused by dental plaque—an adherent film which forms on the teeth as a result of bacterial action. When plaque is more than 24 hours old the bacteria can convert sugar to acid and this acid destroys the enamel of the teeth. Bacterial toxins simultaneously cause gum disease.

The Dental Strategy Review Group was set up by the Department of Health to develop a preventive strategy. Its report, published in 1981, set out a series of measures which were designed to prevent the loss of natural teeth. The measures proposed can be classified under four main headings.

Changes in the physical environment
1 The addition of fluoride to the water supply or, if this is not possible, the provision of fluoride tablets and fluoride toothpaste.
2 The labelling of food to allow foods with sugar to be easily identified.
3 The provision of sugar-free foods in school meals and tuck shops.

Changes in the social environment
1 A more positive attitude to dental health needs to be encouraged; the belief that it is normal to be edentulous by the age of 30 years is now uncommon, but too many people still believe that dental caries and the loss of a few teeth is a normal part of childhood.
2 There is a need to change attitudes towards fluoridation, and

the legal measures that are necessary to introduce it, amongst both the public and politicians.

Health education

There are a number of important dental health education messages.

1 Pregnant women should eat a balanced diet and visit a dentist twice during pregnancy.

2 Tooth brushing should begin as soon as teeth appear and fluoride supplements should be given from 6 months to 12 years of age if there is insufficient in the water.

3 Sugar should not be consumed between meals.

4 Teeth should be adequately brushed at least once a day.

These measures should not be presented in isolation but should be included in general health education programmes and specialist dental health education officers work closely with their colleagues in health education to do this. However, education encouraging self-care is insufficient. The appropriate use of dental services should also be encouraged.

Personal preventive services

The Dental Strategy Review Group not only identified the need for primary prevention, they also identified the need for regular dental inspections. This requires firstly, education of the public to seek help from dentists and dental hygienists, and secondly, the education and organization of the dental profession to increase its emphasis on preventive work. At present the system of payment of dentists discourages preventive work.

These services are important for all people, but they are particularly important for handicapped people. Special services, including dental health education, for the handicapped are organized by community dental officers employed by health authorities to develop a dental strategy, because it is accepted that the general dental practitioner is not able to deliver a satisfactory service to mentally handicapped people or to people living in institutions.

The problems of the edentulous

It might appear that the person who had no natural teeth could not be considered in need of dental disease prevention, but this is not the case. Changes in gum size and structure take place after the teeth have been removed, and people with false teeth have to be taught how to care for both their dentures and their gums and given guidance on when to seek help. Simple advice should be given to elderly people who have no natural teeth, e.g.

1 see your dentist every 2 years or sooner if you have pain or if you notice your dentures becoming loose;

2 keep your dentures in at all times, except at night.

CHAPTER 22

THIRD WORLD HEALTH

The Third World is that part of the earth's population that is neither East nor West, the part that is not concerned with world domination but with survival. The term 'the Third World' has, however, been superseded in recent years by other terms that are sometimes used to describe the poor countries of the world.

The Brandt Commission (the Independent Commission on International Development Issues) discussed two worlds: North and South (Fig. 22.1).

The World Health Organization divides the South, the poorer countries, into two groups: the poorest and the poor (Table 22.1). The poorest countries number about thirty and are found in two poverty belts: one extends across Africa between the Sahara and Lake Nyasa, the other begins with the two Yemens and Afghanistan and stretches across South-east Asia.

Health problems in the Third World

Health statistics in poor countries are often incomplete and in-

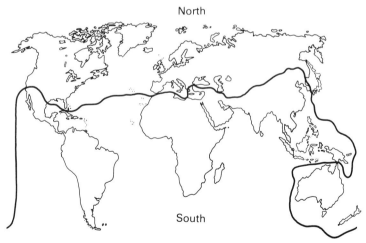

Fig. 22.1. 'North' and 'South': the wealthy countries lie above the line, the poor below it.

Table 22.1 Health and related socio-economic indicators calculated by the WHO*. (After Office of Health Economics (1982) *Health, Medicines and the Poor World.* OHE, London.)

	Least developed countries	Other developing countries	Developed countries
Number of countries	31	89	37
Total population (millions)	283	3 001	1 131
Reported infant mortality rate (per 1000 liveborn)	160	94	19
Life expectancy (years)	45	60	72
% birth weight 2500 g or more	70	83	93
% coverage by safe water supply	31	41	100
% adult literacy rate	28	55	98
Population per doctor	17 000	2 700	520
Population per nurse	6 500	1 500	220
Population per health worker (any type including traditional birth attendant)	2 400	500	130

* Figures in the table are weighted averages, based upon estimates for 1980 or for the latest year for which data are available.

accurate but the principal health problems are strikingly clear:

1 High infant and child mortality rates.

2 Low expectation of life.

3 Childhood mortality dominated by a combination of infection and malnutrition, e.g. 100 million children under the age of 5 years suffer from protein-energy malnutrition, and measles has a 10% mortality where protein-energy malnutrition prevails (when malnutrition is severe measles mortality may be as high as 50%).

4 Adult health is also dominated by infectious diseases (Fig. 22.2): 500 000 people die annually from tuberculosis; 12 million people have leprosy; 200 million people have schistosomiasis; 500 million people have hookworms.

5 Women have higher mortality rates than men: the maternal mortality rate in some countries is 300 times higher than in the U.K.

6 The size of the population is increasing quickly, particularly in those countries in which the infant mortality rate is falling.

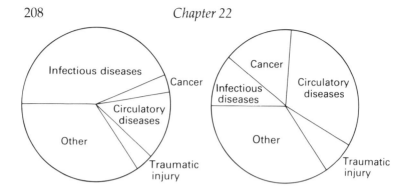

Typical Third World country   Typical industrialized country

Fig. 22.2 Deaths proportioned by cause in the rich and poor countries. (After Office of Health Economics (1982) *Health, Medicines and the Poor World*. OHE, London.)

Causes of health problems

Health problems have to be assessed in the context of other problems. The climate and physical environment of the poorest countries is obviously an important factor but it is inappropriate to ascribe the difference between North and South to these physical differences. Third World countries have a number of social and political characteristics which have to be taken into account when planning preventive services. Not all these factors are present in every poor country and all these characteristics can be identified in the North in developed countries but they are more common in Third World countries.

1 Poverty. Nearly 800 million people live in absolute poverty with insufficient resources to purchase basic requirements.

2 Inequality. In addition to the poverty of the whole country there is marked inequality in many of the poorest countries. Not only is there a large proportion of the population with insufficient money to buy food or with insufficient land on which to grow it but there is also inequality in access to health services and to education.

3 Political instability.

4 An inefficient and, in some countries, corrupt bureaucracy.

5 A low level of literacy and poor means of communication: literacy rates and life expectancy are closely correlated.

6 Inefficient and inappropriate health services.

7 Expenditure of a high proportion of the wealth available for public services on arms.

Health problems cannot be considered in isolation. They are but a part of the problem of poverty. Some people still believe that the problems of people in developing countries are primarily due to the climate and geology of those lands. The infant mortality rate is 160 deaths per 1000 live births in the least developed countries today. However it was 247 per 1000 live births among the more affluent in York in 1898 and the climate and geology of England have not changed significantly in that time. Social and political changes have brought about this fall and are more important than physical factors in determining the health of nations.

Planning preventive services

The prevention of disease requires four types of policy, two of which are general economic policies and two of which are health-service policies.

1 Economic policies to increase wealth.

2 Redistributive policies to redistribute wealth and allow the poorest people access to elementary services.

3 Provision of public health services.

4 Provision of appropriate primary health-care services.

Public health services
Water supply and basic sanitary facilities
One-third of the population of much of Africa and Southern Asia have no access to clean water or sanitary facilities (Fig. 22.3) and 80% of diseases in such areas are caused by water-borne pathogens. About eight million children die every year because of polluted water.

The years 1981–1990 have been designated the UN World Water Decade and progress is being made but because the provision of sewage-disposal systems is less politically attractive than the provision of pure water it seems likely that sewage systems will not be developed so quickly.

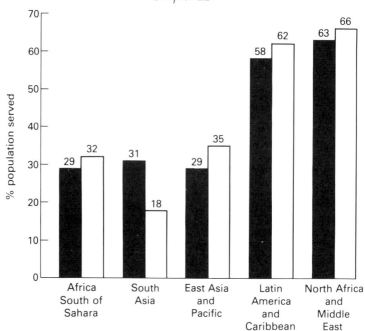

Fig. 22.3. Access to community water supply (■) and excreta disposal services (□) in developing regions. (After World Bank, 1980)

Food

In some poor countries as many as 40% of pre-school children show clinical signs of malnutrition and hundreds of millions of adults suffer from malnutrition. The problem is getting worse as the rate of population growth exceeds the rate of increase of food supply. Some countries which were once self-sufficient now have to import food and as the price of oil increases they have a decreasing amount of money available for the purchase of food. To solve this problem the developing countries must implement the following changes.

1 Increase the amount of land under cultivation, principally by improving irrigation.

2 Use appropriate technology to produce more food per acre.

3 Improve systems of food storage and distribution.

4 Make more use of fish as a source of protein if it is available.

5 Reform inequitable systems of landholding to help the rural poor.

All these steps require assistance from the developed world, in ways that will be discussed in the next section.

Housing
Many people lack secure, safe, warm housing and the problem is being aggravated not only by population growth but also by urbanization; in many countries the major cities are growing at an alarming rate (Table 22.2)

Education
One of the closest correlations is that between life expectancy and literacy (Fig. 22.4). This close correlation does not, of course, mean that reading is a preventive health measure. Literacy rates are a marker of many other aspects of life-style and are a symbol of society's attitudes towards its poorer members. A programme to improve literacy is essential if the health of people in an underdeveloped country is to be improved.

Primary health care services

Many poor countries have health services that are based in hospitals, concentrated in cities, and available to only a small proportion of the population. The WHO convened a conference in Alma-Ata in 1978 and the result of this conference was its commitment to the development of primary health care.

Primary health care, which includes general practice or

Table 22.2 Urbanization rates (After Office of Health Economics (1982) *Health, Medicines and the Poor World*. OHE, London.)

	Estimated population (millions)	
	1975	2000
Mexico City	10.9	31.5
Sao Paulo	9.9	26.0
Cairo	6.9	16.9
Lagos	2.1	9.4
Jakarta	5.6	17.8
Bombay	7.1	19.8

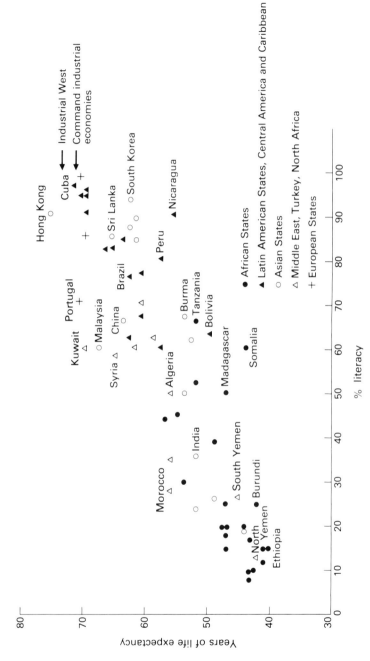

Fig. 22.4. Life expectancy (1979) and literacy in the mid 1970s throughout the world. (After World Bank (1981).)

primary medical care as it is sometimes called, is based on four principles:

1 health services should be planned to meet the needs of the population;

2 the community should participate in the planning of primary health-care services;

3 resources should be used as efficiently as possible;

4 health services should be integrated with other services, e.g. housing and education.

This means that the development of primary health-care services should fit in with the development of other services, such as education, and should be accompanied by economic measures to help those who are least well-off. The objective of the WHO is to ensure 'Health for All by the Year 2000'; the development of relatively inexpensive primary health-care services will play a vitally important part in achieving progress towards this goal.

New challenges for primary health care

Not only have health planners in poor countries to face the problems of infectious diseases, they also have to tackle some of the health risks that affect people in rich countries.

1 Alcohol abuse is an increasing problem in many countries.

2 Cigarette smoking is increasing most quickly in the Third World due largely to the aggressive marketing of the tobacco multinationals.

3 Road-traffic accidents are increasing as the numbers of motor cycles and cars increase.

4 Drug abuse.

Thus, the health minister of a developing country not only has to consider the problems caused by polluted water and malnutrition, he may also have to consider the consequences of an increase in the numbers of people disabled in road-traffic accidents and be prepared to take on the tobacco multinationals.

What can we do?

Give medical aid

Because most doctors and other health professionals are inappropriately trained, it is ineffective simply to give medical services to developing countries unless the contribution that they are going to make has been very carefully considered and tailored to the needs of the individual country. Examples of successful intervention are:

1 the WHO smallpox eradication campaign;
2 provision of medical help in disaster areas by organizations such as Oxfam and the Red Cross;
3 the development of simple, safe, cheap therapies, e.g. the oral rehydration pack for children with diarrhoea by the WHO Diarrhoeal Disease Control Programme.

Give technical and financial aid

The UN suggested that developed countries give 0.7% of their Gross National Product as aid to poor countries but few countries give this degree of help. In 1976 only three of the seventeen richest countries—Norway, Sweden and Holland—gave this and since that time the percentage of GNP that is given as aid by rich countries has declined in many countries.

Furthermore, the aid that some countries give is inappropriate. It is often capital intensive and 'tied' to the donor country; that is the aid given must be spent on goods and services from the donor country, such as a smelter or a factory.

Give opportunities to poor countries

What developing countries need most is opportunity—opportunity to borrow and opportunity to trade. The World Bank can lend money and extend credit but the poorest countries find it more difficult to borrow than those which are better off. There is, however, evidence that this is changing. The World Bank is now more interested in rural, labour-intensive, agricultural projects and is also increasingly interested in encouraging poor countries to consider the needs of their poorest inhabitants.

Poor countries also need the opportunity to trade freely. At present the developed world places a whole series of obstacles in the path of poor countries who wish to trade with them. Scared of the short-term consequences of unemployment and an increase in imports, and unable to grasp or to argue to the electorate the long-term benefits of free trade, politicians resort to protectionism, placing subtle but effective obstacles to the import of products and commodities from the Third World while encouraging free trade within the developed world.

Aid is obviously important to developing countries but the opportunity to borrow and to trade is even more important. Discussions on aid may simply be a salve for our conscience because we in the developed world are not prepared to allow poor countries freedom to trade.

Divert resources to health

Although developed countries have economic problems they are very wealthy and one of the reasons that so little of that wealth is spent on health is that so much is spent on arms. In many developing countries arms expenditure dominates government spending, to an even greater degree than in the developed world. The Brandt Report (1980 *North–South: A Programme for Survival.* The Report of the Independent Commission on International Issues under the Chairmanship of Willy Brandt) spelled out the costs and consequences of arms expenditure very clearly:

1 The military expenditure of only half a day would suffice to finance the whole malaria eradication programme of the WHO, and less would be needed to conquer river-blindness, which is still the scourge of millions.

2 A modern tank costs about one million dollars; that amount could improve storage facilities for 100 000 tons of rice and thus save 4000 tons or more annually: one person can live on just over a pound of rice a day. The same sum of money could provide 1000 classrooms for 30 000 children.

3 For the price of one jet fighter (20 million dollars) one could set up about 40 000 village pharmacies.

4 One-half of 1% of one year's world military expenditure would pay for all the farm equipment needed to increase food production and approach self-sufficiency in food-deficit, low-income countries by 1990.

What can I do?

Hundreds of millions suffering from preventable diseases; millions of children dying from preventable causes; hundreds of millions of pounds needed for primary health care—what can an individual do? The answer is more than he thinks. He can:

1 Give financial support to a charity working in the Third World; 0.7% of his GNP, his annual salary, is a good target (£70 pa or £6 per month for someone with a salary of £10 000).

2 Be well-informed and able to counter ill-informed statements about the problems of the Third World.

3 Offer his technical expertise if it is relevant.

4 Write to his MP when major reports on Third World health are produced or when aid is discussed in Parliament.

This may not seem much but if even 10% of the electorate supported it the effect would be considerable.

FURTHER READING

Plagues and Peoples by W. H. McNeil (Blackwell 1977) is a fascinating account of the factors which have influenced the epidemics of infectious disease, and in *The Role of Medicine* (Blackwell 1979) Thomas McKeown considers the decline of infectious disease in nineteenth century Britain in more detail. Chapter 6 of *Man Against Disease* by Muir Gray (Oxford University Press 1979) discusses the politics of prevention and Lord Ashby's book *Reconciling Man with the Environment* (Oxford University Press 1978) provides some interesting case studies. *Preventive Medicine in General Practice* by Muir Gray and Godfrey Fowler (Oxford University Press 1983) describes preventive health services, with a particular emphasis on the work of the general practitioner.

The Royal College of General Practitioners have produced a useful series of discussion papers which focus on the potential for prevention in general practice:

- Family planning—an exercise in preventive medicine (RCGP 1981);
- Healthier children—thinking prevention (RCGP 1981);
- Prevention of arterial disease in general practice (RCGP 1982);
- Prevention of psychiatric disorders in general practice (RCGP 1981);
- Promoting prevention (RCGP 1983).

Antenatal and Neonatal Screening, edited by N. J. Wald (Oxford University Press 1983) is an excellent reference book.

Child Health by Aidan Macfarlane summarizes the steps that can be taken to prevent illness in childhood and adolescence, and *Geriatric Problems in General Practice* (Oxford University Press) by Gordon Wilcock, Muir Gray and Peter Pritchard, the scope for prevention in old age.

Exercise—the Facts by Peter Fentem and Joan Bassey (Oxford University Press 1980) is a good review of the beneficial effects of exercise.

Inequalities in Health by Peter Townsend and Nick Davidson is a published version of a Government Report which analyses the causes of social class differences in health and suggests ways in which these may be overcome. The Department of Health has produced a useful series of bookets—Prevention and Health, everybody's business (HMSO)—on the common preventable causes of death:

- Occupational Health Services (HMSO 1977);
- Pattern and range of services for problem drinkers (HMSO 1978);
- Eating for health (HMSO 1978);
- Prevention in the child health services (HMSO 1980);
- Avoiding heart attacks (HMSO 1981);
- Drinking sensibly (HMSO 1981);
- Towards better dental health—guidelines for the future (HMSO 1981).

Other useful Government papers are the Report of the House of Commons Expenditure Committee on Preventive Medicine (HMSO 1977) and the White Paper on Prevention and Health (HMSO 1977).

The health hazards of smoking are summarized in the Report of the Royal College of Physicians: *Health or Smoking* (Pitman 1983). In addition the reports of the U.S. Surgeon General, notably *Smoking and Health* (U.S. Department of Health Education and Welfare 1979).

The scope for prevention of cancer is lucidly summarized in *The Causes of Cancer* by Richard Doll and Richard Peto (Oxford University Press 1981) and the problems of the Third World by the report of the Independent Commission on International Development Issues—the Brandt Report, which has been published as *North South: A Programme for Survival* (Pan 1980).

INDEX

219